Close to Me,
But Far Away

Close to Me, But Far Away

LIVING WITH ALZHEIMER'S

Burton M. Wheeler

University of Missouri Press

Columbia and London

Cataloging-in-Publication Data available from the Library of
Congress. ISBN 0-8262-1380-4

⊗ This paper meets the requirements of the
American National Standard for Permanence of Paper
for Printed Library Materials, Z39.48, 1984.

Text designer: Elizabeth K. Young
Cover designer: Susan Ferber
Typesetter: The Composing Room of Michigan, Inc.
Printer and binder: Thomson-Shore, Inc.
Typefaces: Stone Sans Semibold, Stone Informal (Regular)

Quotation from T. S. Eliot's "Little Gidding" used with the kind
permission of Valerie Eliot and Faber and Faber Ltd.

Dedicated to the Alzheimer's Association
and Its More than 150 Local Chapters

Close to Me,
But Far Away

We live beneath canopies: the canopy of trees, luxuriant in spring, brown and naked in winter; the canopy of the heavens, blindingly bright, terrifyingly dark, often merely gray. There are canopies we fashion for ourselves, awkwardly copied from the patterns we choose and frayed by time. We live under these canopies because, to claim life fully, we must.

I have a pedestrian mind. Some people soar to pinnacles of revelation, and others leap abysses to arrive at unshakable conclusions, but I just plod along. As I struggle through tangles of undergrowth that constrict my vision, I try to be attentive to whatever I can observe, but I often stumble, and my hesitant pace leads to a shortsighted, quizzical outlook. Frankly, I accept this quality as useful to my new vocation.

My new vocation is that of caregiver. I didn't choose the vocation or the term. Both were thrust upon me. A vocation is not a choice; it is a calling, one to which I responded before I knew what it was. You know the feeling. Things develop at their own pace, quietly, surreptitiously, until one day you discover that you are immersed in an unexpected role. You've been performing the tasks of caregiver before you are aware of the summons. We either heed the call or struggle frantically, trying to pretend that the summons wasn't all that clear. I'm no Jacob. I don't have the stamina to wrestle with an angel.

My wife has Alzheimer-type dementia. According to one study, there are four million sufferers of this fate in the United States alone. By my count that means another twelve to sixteen million are to some degree caregivers. My misery doesn't enjoy company, but there it is.

Why am I uncomfortable with the term *caregiver?* It implies to me a constancy and stability of which I am incapable. The term sounds static—a steady state of devoted performance. I wish I were capable of such behavior, but I'm not. My moods fluctuate wildly. Some days I awake and rush energetically to my daily chores—cleaning and changing my wife, washing, drying, and putting away clothes, towels, and sheets, preparing meals, feeding my wife, putting her back to bed, changing her, getting her up again, working on budgets in which categories seep and ooze into one another—relying on aides so that I can shop, pick up medications, and occasionally escape for

1

the exercise I must have to survive. Actually I've never made it through an entire day with such a rush of energy. When I reach the finish line, about eleven P.M., I'm short of breath, and my eyes roll toward the back of my head.

Most mornings I crawl out of bed slowly. Not only slowly, but painfully. I'm in my mid-seventies. Not one muscle, not one bone fails to protest the necessity of getting up. I try not to think about anything until I've had my coffee, preferably two cups. My mind has to go through its own gymnastic routines before it will function. Those routines demand caffeine.

The diagnosis "Alzheimer-type dementia" is a convenient shorthand. No one knows with absolute certainty whether my wife has the disease and won't know until an autopsy is performed after her death. Yes, there will be an autopsy in the hope that any knowledge gained will be useful in the continuing study directed toward eliminating the disease or at least lessening its destructiveness. What will the pathologists find? Plaques and tangles, of course, things which have destroyed the normal functioning of one I love. They will not find what I have lost.

I and the twelve to sixteen million like me are operating on an assumption. Neurologists assure us that current evidence indicates that approximately 93 percent of competent diagnoses of Alzheimer-type dementia are proven accurate by autopsy. (Did you catch those weasel words? *Current* and *competent* send up red flares: "We may be wrong about this!")

By now you know that I can be crabby and suspicious. I would be lying if I said I'm at peace with the world. Having a pedestrian mind doesn't mean I'm dull-witted, just that I've learned to be cautious, to consider no evidence conclusive. Early in my new vocation I realized that if I could avoid all thought I could probably perform my perfunctory, daily routines better. Life would be easier if my intellect and imagination could be sealed up behind drywall. Then I could quit asking constantly: "What if . . . ?" But I can't, nor, I suspect, can my fellow sufferers. In fact, I do not wish to surrender thought, imagination, or memory, for those are the qualities—the human qualities—stripped from my wife. Alzheimer's disease. It will win the war, but I want to throw my puny strength into every struggle, every skirmish.

Some people in the Alzheimer's circle don't like the term *victim*, I'm told. When I first heard that, I thought I was in a strange land with an alien language. I sure *think* I'm a victim, and I'm absolutely certain my wife is, although she doesn't worry about it. For that I'm grateful. But, do I really know what she thinks? Does anyone know what goes on in the mind of an Alzheimer's patient?

Anyway, this is my story, or rather, our story. The woman I love and with whom I've shared life for fifty years began about nine or ten years ago to sink into a swamp from which I could not save her. Sometimes I think that if I could only pinpoint when her illness began, I could understand her needs better. Why it began is a question I try not to ask; I don't wish to enter that frightening realm of mystery. But it might help to know when. A paleontologist could excavate old bones and from them conceptualize what role those bones played on their stage. But I only disinter memories and am no longer confident of the accuracy of what I recall.

I can't even explain why understanding the beginning of my wife's dementia is so important; it just is. Beginning, middle, end—a logical conception, a dramatic necessity, but I can only comprehend middle. For the beginning I can identify no single symptom, no moment of contagion, no distinctive act. There was no evident trigger, no first domino—only sequence, middle, time sliding through time. Yet there had to be a beginning. Because I can't find it, I sometimes want to fabricate it. Genesis: "In the beginning. . . ." Out of chaos I want to create beginning. But chaos already was, and had no beginning.

Before a doctor used the word *Alzheimer,* we feared that diagnosis. Initially, I refused to believe my wife was suffering from dementia. Something was wrong, yes, but she was too perceptive, too alert for such an illness. What was wrong I didn't know, but the "what" seemed less important than getting her back to normal. Gradually each day simply faded into another. Each week, each month into yet another. There was no beginning, no end, only continuity of time. The burden of day following day sometimes seemed unbearable.

I can remember many of the details of what seemed at the time to be depression. She became listless; the brightness of her eyes dimmed. She lost interest in going to concerts, plays, movies. Her enthusiasm for travel vanished. I dug up maps and dragged down books trying to stimulate her interest in what we had long wanted to do—make a trip to Greece and the Cyclades Islands. Nothing worked.

That she was tired was not surprising. Her days were often long. Some days she was in her office from eight A.M. to eight P.M., adjusting her hours to meet the schedules of her patients. No psychotherapist was ever more committed to those who sought help. Our vacations were usually short because she did not want to be away from her clients for prolonged periods. Even weekends were sometimes sacrificed to their needs.

Gradually I took over the shopping, cooking, and gardening chores. With our children grown and involved with their own lives, those tasks were not onerous. As I moved toward retirement, I had more time. Simultaneously, her work became increasingly demanding. In a small way I felt I was repaying her for the many years she had done most of those tasks. But her exhaustion troubled me. Was she just working too hard? How could I help? I began driving her to her office and picking her up whenever she was ready to return home.

Stories in newspapers and magazines suggested an explanation. "Chronic fatigue" was the illness of the day. As articles proliferated and anecdotes of sufferers became common, there was no way I could ignore that possibility. When I proposed this diagnosis to her physician, he was not impressed. But in a rigorous physical examination, he found a tumor in her right breast.

She told no one beyond the immediate family that she was to have a mastectomy. Everything had to be subordinate to the well-being of her patients. She did not want them to know. I delayed making any more plans for Greece. During a "vacation" (allegedly we were out of town), she underwent surgery, then returned to her patients in less than a month. Because my relationship to students bore the same stamp of commitment, I understood. Certainly I supported her devotion to her work.

As far as I could tell, she dealt with the loss of her breast and the reconstructive surgery as well as one can. She didn't like to talk about it, but I did all that I knew how to do to make her feel comfortable. I praised her appearance, and we continued to have intercourse, tender and loving. Yet neither of us could pretend there was no change. One evening as we talked she broke out in an angry attack on the surgeon. She declared that he had botched the rebuilding of her breast. Yes, there was extensive scar tissue, but she had always scarred easily. And yes, the breast sagged badly, but we were assured that the tumor had been successfully removed; neither chemotherapy nor radiation was required. She continued to insist that the surgeon had done a terrible job.

Her fatigue worsened. The threat of other cancers was constantly in her thoughts. She feared that an undetected tumor was metastasizing, that her body was slowly being ravaged by cancer. I assured her that all tests indicated otherwise and suggested that her depression might be related to the sudden death of her mother several years earlier, she denied any connection. She did not deny that she was depressed. Mistakenly, I attributed all her changes in behavior to depression.

As her depression deepened, I encouraged her to return to the psychoanalyst with whom she had worked a decade earlier. She did but quite suddenly broke off the relationship, saying the analyst wasn't supportive enough. She began to talk about death more frequently.

Quite imperceptibly to those of us blinded by the ferocity of our love and by our urgent need for her to behave as we wanted and expected, she quit reading. Only later did I realize that books taken on trips went unopened. Professional journals piled up without covers removed. Whether by rational processes or by intuition, she had, I now believe, discovered that her mind could neither process nor retain new information. Perhaps she also discovered how easily she could conceal this loss from others, including me. In many respects, she seemed normal, unchanged. Her attentive expression, her understanding nod of approval, a smile at the appropriate moment, and none of us who loved her could know what she knew. Colleagues, clients, and acquaintances noticed nothing. They were so accustomed to her warmth and graciousness that they were oblivious to her failing memory.

Later it occurred to me that Alzheimer-type dementia does its insidious work as quietly and destructively as termites. It eats away at the core, leaving the surface seemingly intact. Before the damage is recognized, it is irreversible.

Using her weariness as an excuse, she decided to retire. After giving up her office and work, and the clients to whom she was so dedicated, she spent most of her days in bed, sometimes napping, but more often lying there with unfocused eyes.

I concocted excuses to get her out of the house. I used ruses to get her to take walks with me. I took her to movies I did not want to see. And we left early from some of those I did want to see. We went out to dinner more frequently. When I had to make a trip, fearful of leaving her alone, I arranged for her to accompany me. She was usually cooperative, pleasantly doing whatever I asked or suggested. She even seemed to enjoy some of the things we did and places we went, but there were no lasting benefits. On trips out of town she became more and more inclined to stay in hotel rooms when I had meetings.

Looking back, I ask myself if I was engaging in manipulative behavior. Probably. But then I ask what else I could have done. It was impossible for me to give up trying to do something.

Our children also suggested ways to develop new interests, but none of their suggestions worked either. I became aware of my increasing irritability. Thinking it was important to conceal this growing anger and impatience, I unconsciously began to repress my feelings, knowing nevertheless that rage was mounting and becoming more flammable. On long walks by myself, I struggled to confront anger and the deep-seated fear that I was inadequate to the task of dealing with whatever illness possessed her.

She could not articulate her fears. Neither I nor our children could imagine them. She turned to more alcohol, an extra glass or two of wine, more than her small body could manage. Even in pregnancy she had never weighed more than 125 pounds. Now at less than 110 pounds, she slurred her speech and moved sluggishly whenever she had more than one drink. Seeking relief in the numbing effects of alcohol, she inadvertently gave us a reasonable, if mistaken, explanation for her behavior. When the children, now in their thirties and forties, came home for holidays, they scolded her. They and I held her accountable and warned of impending consequences. For several years we continued to confuse symptoms with causes, unable to recognize what was happening to her mind. We simply did not recognize that alcohol was but one of her efforts to conceal from herself, as well as others, her awareness that she was slowly losing her powers of perception and rationality.

Focusing on our concern about her drinking, the children and I overlooked her forgetfulness about schedules or trivia recently introduced in conversation. One night she told the same story—a story drawn from her experience running a day care center—three times within two hours to dinner guests, and I attributed it to her having had several glasses of wine. Seizing upon my fears that she was becoming an alcoholic, I cleared all alcoholic beverages out of the house and kept them out for over a year. There was no improvement.

The children and I became as adept at avoiding the reality of her illness as she had become. Possibly we put on blinders because we did not want to know the truth. To confront dementia demanded more than we could bear. The truth threatened to scald our too-tender sensibilities, leaving raw flesh and agonizing pain.

Not until much later, after reading *The 36-Hour Day* and coming to understand more about the development of Alzheimer-type dementia, did I recognize a pattern of behavior that almost certainly was an early symptom of the disease. I can't remember just when the first incident occurred, but it must have been about the time of her mastectomy. One day, quite unexpectedly, she announced her bitter dislike of a friend. Taken aback, I said, "But you've always liked her. You've enjoyed being with her." Her response was irritable, irrational. I let the matter drop.

Not long thereafter, a misunderstanding arose with a group of lay counselors whom she had been training. She now felt that persons with whom she had long worked cooperatively and constructively were unsupportive, even hostile. She provoked an incident that led to further misunderstandings. I tried to get her to explain why she felt as she did. She would not discuss the matter with me; it was none of my business. Finally, she simply withdrew from the group, giving no adequate explanation to anyone. She was both inflicting and receiving wounds, but I could not recognize her anger for what it was.

One day she received a letter from a cousin reporting the death of a more distant cousin. She blurted out, "May he rot in Hell!" Such an outburst was stunningly uncharacteristic of my gentle wife. All I could say was "Why?" Angrily she described the cousin's molesting her when she was nine. With even greater anger she described her parents' disbelief and unwillingness to confront the boy or his parents. That the incident was deeply painful and had gained power from its long repression, I recognized, but the passion with which she denounced her parents and consigned the dead cousin to hell was not like her. But again, she refused to discuss it further, retreating into a private world. All I could say was something rather lame like "I'm not surprised that you hated him." Yet I was disturbed by the intensity she expressed.

Over the next several years she dug up several incidents from the past, reliving them and cultivating her anger. Outbursts were directed against her dead mother, against living relatives, against cherished friends. I found it troubling, even frightening, but I did not recognize a pattern. She had always been "slow to anger" unless one of her children was endangered. And her expressions of anger toward me had been far less frequent than I deserved.

Then an incident occurred I could not ignore. One night, one of our sons telephoned. I answered the phone, we talked briefly, and then he asked to speak to his mother, who was in another room. I called out that her son wanted to talk with her, but she refused to answer. Thinking she might not have understood, I went to get her. She said, "I don't ever want to talk to him again." I was stunned. Returning to the phone, I lied, telling our son that his mother couldn't come to the phone but would call him soon. After hanging up, I confronted her: "Why don't you want to talk to him?" She said, "He doesn't love me. He didn't call me on Mother's Day!" Mother's Day was yet ten days away.

Two years later, after reading in *The 36-Hour Day* that Alzheimer's victims sometimes suffer from paranoia, I came to think that her anger over grievances—real and imagined—was the earliest clinical evidence of her deterioration. Since I, alone, observed the frequency of her anger, only I could have recognized that there was a pattern, but I was unfamiliar with dementia, protective of her, and lost in a fog of denial.

Her confusion about time made any resentment current. An old, half-forgotten slight became a present source of pain. It was her unjustified anger at our son that finally moved me to insist on a psychiatric examination. I doubted that my observations were sound, but I felt I had to have help. Looking back, I suspect my fear of the diagnosis prevented me from seeking professional help earlier. Now it seems so straightforwardly necessary, but seven years ago I felt deeply guilty both for making the appointment and insisting that she go. I promised to drive her, to stay with her, and return home with her.

After seeing her alone, the psychiatrist, whom we both knew, invited me to join them in his office. Offering no diagnosis, he suggested that we go to a specialist in geriatric psychiatry, someone Kee had never met. Initially, she balked at accepting the referral, but I begged her to go, insisted that she go, and when she finally consented, was surprised that she agreed. What would I have done had she refused? I really don't know.

After the first meeting with the new doctor, she even agreed to undergo an extensive battery of tests given by a clinical psychologist. After the tests and several visits to the specialist, the dreaded sentence was pronounced: "Alzheimer-type dementia." Oh, it wasn't that blunt. The doctor was considerate and sensitive, but he knew that we saw him as virtually a "hanging judge" if not an executioner.

I cannot recall any details of our drive home. We were not in shock. We had heard what at one level of understanding we had both expected and feared, but we had also hoped for a diagnosis that left some hope. The finality of the sentence drove us both deep into our own feelings. Whatever we said to one another was intended to be mutually reassuring, but our words were no more substantive than dust.

Subsequently I met with the psychiatrist alone. What I recall most vividly from that meeting was my wife's appallingly low score on a standard intelligence test. Her score was barely over 50 percent of what it had been years earlier.

As the certainty of the diagnosis pressed upon me, I fluctuated between fear that I could not possibly manage and the awareness that I had to. There was no point of equilibrium. Like a yo-yo, I spun up and down, reacting to the slightest tug. In a moment of confidence, I inexplicably broke into tears. Knowing that self-pity would destroy me, I tried to fight it, but even now I have not completely freed myself from its tentacles. For me that is a painful admission.

I said before that I dislike the term *caregiver*. The word seems to lump us all together. We are each distinctive. And certainly we are not proverbial angels of mercy. We bring to our relationships and labors diverse anxieties and fears. We are committed to attending to the ones we love, but we want our full humanity to be recognized. And because we are, I think, painfully conscious of our flaws and failures, we are often moody and unpredictable. We cannot go it alone, yet our needs are contradictory. We want support and love; we want to be left alone. To tell you that I am a caregiver tells you only how I spend much of my time.

The same problem, of course, exists with names. My friends call me Burt. Does that help? Names designate, but they also give an illusion of understanding. I am multiple Burts—angry and joyful, idealistic and cynical, hopeful and hopeless, defiant and acquiescent. In short, I find myself caught in multiple roles. At times I want to strike out maliciously, but I also love, deeply love, an invalid wife. Sometimes I simply feel tired, tired of everything. So who am I? Perhaps we are quite alike, you and I.

My wife's given name is Jacquelyn, but she has always been called Jackie. As I try to express what this past decade has been like, I find that, in telling you our story, I cannot use her name. The name represents who she was before her dementia invaded. Her maiden name ended with the same syllable as Jackie, and I sometimes playfully called her by that final syllable—Kee. In telling our story, I have chosen to use that abbreviated, attenuated name. Her life, too, is attenuated. I do not love her less, but who Jackie was is not who she is, at least not completely. Perhaps, too, I am pretending that, by calling her Kee, I will not embarrass her.

Several years ago, in the early stages of my wife's dementia, I discovered that I was far more weary and depressed than I had admitted. I had been so busy trying to be heroic and omni-competent that I had lost touch with myself. Repression had become a principal characteristic of my life—repression of anger, repression of resentment, repression of that healthy selfishness which speaks to one's own need for physical and emotional survival. I set out to try to gain some distance from being me by trying to observe what I was doing day in and day out, hour by hour, and writing about what I saw. Call it self-inflicted therapy.

After a year or so, I showed what I had written to my children and a few friends. They thought others should read it. Then I shared it with more friends, considering how I felt about revealing quite private facets of our lives. To share our story is not easy, and I sometimes feel that because I do not have my wife's consent, I am betraying her. To tell the full story, the true story, I must be frank. I must pull back curtains normally closed, violating a privacy which is her right and which I want to honor.

With the aid of our children, I concluded that, if my companion, my dearest friend, were fully cognizant, she would indeed be deeply embarrassed by many of the details. So am I. But with the support of our children I decided that Jackie would have wanted to make this story public if it could in any way help others. Her life has been a testimony to truth and caring.

Unlike most human ailments, Alzheimer-type dementia is unaccompanied by pain. The agony of cancer or MLS or ALS (Lou Gehrig's disease) is entirely missing. For the caregiver, however, psychological distress leading to physical discomfort is common. We may experience acute pain from shingles or migraines or live with steady, unnerving, nagging aches from muscles and joints strained by our actions.

When I assert that Kee is essentially free of pain, that I am the one who suffers, why should you believe me? I hope by now you are eager to hear Kee's voice, what she has been thinking and feeling these last six or seven years. Sadly, I cannot provide that voice, nor can she. Regrettably, our story must be told as a monologue.

Monologues are difficult to authenticate, and I distrust them. In life, as in the theater, we need other persons and voices to establish the ground of reality, the truthfulness of any speaker. Perhaps Kee no longer realizes that this is a story, a drama, a playing out of two lives. Dialogue, the sharing of thoughts, has disappeared. Only one voice— that of a confused, often disheartened, but still determined husband of one who has been victimized by Alzheimer's disease—can tell our story now.

In telling our story, I can describe our experiences only from my understanding. Kee cannot help us understand whatever she is experiencing. Nevertheless, she is the center of my life. What I do, what I think, how I feel—all these things are influenced by the person she remains. That an intelligence which has mysteriously disappeared could make many things clearer, perhaps even easier, adds to the distress I feel.

The physical pain suffered by caregivers is, I think, less severe than what I can only call the pain of the heart: the agony of what might have been, the anguish of regret. Kee was diagnosed with AD in late 1994. Our grandson, Cody, was born in early January 1993. When

Kee's diagnosis was made, the doctors believed that she had already reached the middle stages of the disease. At the time Cody was conceived in 1992, dementia was already incubating in Kee. Our grandson's new life—vibrant, pulsing, his mind eagerly absorbing all that his senses encounter—distressingly counterpoints the gradual decay of Kee's intelligence. Forced to observe the development of my grandson against Kee's slow deterioration to an infantile state has been devastating. But perhaps my best defense against self-pity and surrender arises from his vitality. He whirls into the house like a gale-force wind. No visit is quite like any other.

Like everything else in life, being a grandparent is a role, although a distinctive one. I even have my own name in the play—Grumps. When Kristin, our daughter, and her husband asked what we would like to be called, Kee chose Ya-Ya, Greek for grandmother. That was two years before the AD diagnosis.

Before our daughter was born, we lived above a woman in her seventies who had immigrated from Greece as a young woman. Her accent charmed our two boys; her generosity charmed us all. She gave Kee lessons in rolling out the thin sheets of pastry used for baklava and spinach pie and plied the children with lollipops. "Please Ya-Ya," Kee said, "don't give them so much candy." "They need candy," Ya-Ya replied. "Well," said Kee, "just give them one each." Ya-Ya, handing out two lollipops to each boy, responded, "I should like one hand better than the other?" Ya-Ya embodied all that is good in grandmothering.

I couldn't think of an exotic name to be called. I considered "Gramps" but then was intrigued with the possibilities existing in "Grumps." That, I thought, would give me more latitude. Grumps I became. I know that my grandson has difficulty with the name and will until he becomes older, but by the time he is a teenager, he might appreciate my choice. He likely will also think it apt. I'm not sure how long I can maintain a playful outlook while struggling with the fact that I am often tired and grumpy.

That summary is merely a preface to saying that the greatest tragedy arising from Kee's illness is neither her affliction nor mine. By the time our grandson was three, Kee could no longer relate to the child. She could not enjoy his coming. His constant activity and the loud noises that accompanied it befuddled her. Increasingly she became remote when he was present. By the time the boy was four, he was ignoring Kee, expressing overt hostility, or complaining about my attention to her. I believe I understand why. When I was six or seven, I encountered a child with Down's syndrome. I became frightened and distraught. My distress couldn't be articulated nor my fears explained. Now when my grandson says, "I don't like Ya-Ya," I know she frightens him, not by anything she does but by her unresponsiveness and vacant air. I've tried to reassure the boy, but know his distress is real and know that he will not overcome it until he matures. Each needs the other, and I desperately want them to relate well—as they would have, had AD not entered our lives.

I am absolutely certain Kee would have been a wonderful grandmother. Now our grandson, through no fault of his own, can never know what he has been denied. For the remainder of my life, this loss will be a sorrow I cannot overcome. I can imagine no way to give the child more than a glimpse of the love, the generosity, and the extraordinary sensitivity and warmth that characterized his grandmother before her illness. Such is the anguish of regret.

Let me warn you about our story. It does not, it cannot have a happy ending. And I will not shrink from confronting feelings and situations omitted from much of the popular writing about Alzheimer's.

What I experience is, I think, common to other spouses and children who serve as primary caregivers. What I will describe necessarily focuses on the caregiver's life—its volatility, its constant readjusting to things both mundanely practical and psychologically intangible. I say necessarily because no one can fathom the life of the primary victim of Alzheimer's dementia, and we have to learn not to trust the inferences we too readily draw. There was a time when I knew no one as well as I knew Kee. Now there is no one about whom I am less certain. Experience has taught me that I cannot trust her language and that I may misconstrue the cues of her body language because of my own needs. What I know is who she was. What sustains me are those memories. What drives me on is both the desire to serve her as she is and the need to understand myself in this new and unanticipated relationship. We have both changed; we are both changing.

To conceal either unpleasantness or exhaustion, to pretend that it is a pleasure and privilege for a caregiver to try to decipher the victim's new behavior or to clean up adult feces, is deceptive, dishonest. The only reason I don't call what I have written the "unvarnished truth" is because there are too many truths about the scourge of Alzheimer's.

Ahead of you lies one of my days, a day much like any other, full of nonglorious events which pile up willy-nilly like dirty clothes. The caregiver reacts to and reflects on these events, struggling to understand and wavering between tears and laughter, for the caregiver is both actor and observer. The earthbound details of the experience are intensified for us because we know and fear what our future holds. The essential purpose of our lives has become survival—surviving to care for the afflicted ones we love. What will happen? How will we manage when purpose disappears?

A caregiver is, I think, a bit like a lone passenger on a plane caught in heavy turbulence. He or she cannot control the sudden, stomach-wrenching drops or the shuddering of the fuselage as the plane is buffeted by storms. The pilot or attendant may offer soothing words or clean up spilled coffee, but the passenger who survives such an ordeal will relive the experience over and over—alone.

I don't know any caregiver who wants to change places with the afflicted, but we cannot avoid resenting the ceaseless demands of time and place to which our loved ones are altogether oblivious. All the physical and emotional needs of the afflicted demand immediate attention. My own life becomes more and more restricted. My friendships are stressed because I can no longer cultivate them; my energy is reduced and easily consumed; whatever constructive imagination I had is stunted. Time is a burden. I am a caregiver.

To fulfill my vocation as caregiver, I know I must survive, physically and emotionally. The qualities necessary to that survival begin with deep affection for my wife as she was, as she is, even as she may become. Almost equally important are stamina, adaptability, stubbornness (call it courage, if you prefer, but I think it's mule-headed obstinacy, a sort of "I will not be licked" attitude), and humor, the ability to step back and laugh at the absurdity of so many situations. These qualities lessen the suffering. Nothing eliminates it.

Those of us who are primary caregivers live our lives one day at a time, and each day is a reliving of what has passed before and will likely occur on the morrow. We plod along, sometimes missing the forest, I suppose, but conscious of every individual tree and particularly aware of the briars and brambles where we spend much of our time. To deny the reality of the pain, the difficulty of maintaining physical and emotional health, and the inevitability of our defeat in the struggle to maintain life is absurd. It's also destructive.

Those of us who have accepted our caregiving vocations have willingly—but please, please, not gladly—surrendered the lives we once dreamed of. If you continue reading this, be of good cheer—whenever you can. There is modest satisfaction in knowing that other caregivers know and share our experiences. We form an aggrieved community and the Alzheimer's Association, nationally and locally, eagerly offers help whenever it can. My advice is their advice: Keep putting one foot in front of the other, again and again and again. Unfortunately, that act is more difficult than it sounds. There are moments when "Why?" intrudes, moments when the mere act of moving one foot forward requires all the strength one can summon.

Come along. Here is one of my memorable days, memorable because it is like all the rest. I'll try to make it coherent for you, but I will necessarily fail. There is no tidy coherence in the lives of caregivers. Unlike the sufferers we care for, we retain habits of mind that drive us toward unanswerable questions. We retain memories, vital and satisfying memories, which help us trudge through the days. And those same memories summon up inexplicable sadness because they remind us of different, lost relationships.

Consciousness creeps through me as slowly as shadows form at dawn. I'm aware that I'm not asleep, but my body is indifferent to the waking state. After what may be only a few seconds, I raise my arms and stretch. My eyes focus gradually on the canopy stretched over our old tester bed. The mistakes made by my mother-in-law when she crocheted it fascinate me morning after morning. Again I count them. There are twelve, but I only locate eleven. The orderliness of the geometric pattern usually causes each missed stitch to call attention to itself. I wonder if stitch is the proper word for crocheting.

My mother-in-law was a good woman, and because the crocheting of the canopy was an act of love, or at least affection, I never said anything to her about the mistakes. Nor did she ever suggest there were any. Kee is the only other person who shares this view of the canopy—lying five feet below—seeing it silhouetted against the ceiling. Kee has never understood my preoccupation with the flaws. I think she suspects that my attention to the errors arises from some resentment of my mother-in-law, but it doesn't. For whatever reason, I am compelled to notice such errors, to contemplate failed symmetry, and to wish I knew how to perfect the pattern.

I rise on one elbow and look at Kee sleeping beside me. Her legs angle toward the corner of my side of the bed. Probably some movement of her legs woke me, but it's time to get up. Why? No reason. It's just time to get up. I might as well start the day.

Since her illness began, Kee has slept to my left because that side is closer to the bathroom and there is more room for the wheelchair. Before the coming of Alzheimer's, our positions in bed were reversed because we found sharing love physically more satisfying if I were on my right side and she on her left. For the last few years, only the quest for ease, safety, and a good night's sleep have shaped our sleeping habits.

Usually we shared the bedclothes equitably, but now, in her turning, she often twists them beneath her. When I am not in bed with her, I tuck the upper sheet in as far as I can on both sides to prevent her wrapping up in the sheets and getting them wet. When I am in bed with her, I use my body to pin down the sheets and to keep her on the pad that protects the mattress. Kee has the habit of gradually inching toward my side of the bed. Maybe she needs to feel close, but sometimes her hair in my face or an elbow in my ribs wakes me. She usually responds to a gentle nudge, but there are nights when I climb out of bed, pull out a futon I keep under the bed for our grandson, and sleep on it.

We've never wanted twin beds. And anyway, years ago, when we slept in queen- or king-sized beds in motels and hotels, we usually awakened to find our bodies entwined in one corner of the bed. Now, if I don't have freedom of movement, I have difficulty sleeping.

Though spacious by normal standards, our bedroom seems shrunken by the massive furniture we brought here when we sold our home. Our tester bed is about eight feet high and longer than a standard bed. Our walnut armoire with Jacobean decoration matching that of the bedposts is even larger. Kee purchased the old bed, probably mid-nineteenth century, at an auction. Two years later she found the armoire. They matched so well that she ignored my warning that the two pieces together were too large and that there was only one windowless wall in our house that could take an armoire about eight feet by nine feet. When Kee liked a piece, she was very, very convincing. We bought it.

When we sold the house where we had lived for fifteen years, her one condition was that we find a condominium large enough to hold the bedroom furniture. The moment we entered this building with its high ceiling and windows overlooking the park, we knew it was right for us. We made the move just in time; two years later would have been too late.

Kee is still asleep, breathing heavily, but undisturbed by my movements. I swing both legs over the side of the bed carefully and pull myself into a sitting position, pausing for a few moments to gather wits and balance. I no longer have instinctive confidence in either. I'm not really old, I suppose, but I certainly feel old, especially in the early morning. The last ten years have taken a heavy toll on my self-confidence, both physical and mental.

The alarm clock on the bedside table says 6:58. I no longer set the alarm because I usually awaken around 7:00 and since I retired there is no reason to get up earlier. Even if we oversleep, nothing is lost. I keep the time set correctly because the digital glow at night enables me to monitor how much time my bladder allows me between trips to the bathroom. Last night I went to the bathroom only twice, bouncing off door facings and steadying myself against the sink, of course, but only twice.

Now, half awake, I limp out of the bedroom, away from its bathroom, and down the hall toward my bathroom, the one just off my study. My walking is improving, but in the early morning a limp still troubles me. I am limping because three months ago I failed to get my feet in the proper position when I was moving Kee from her wheelchair into bed. Twisting my body while holding all of her weight in my arms damaged the nerves controlling my left leg. Within two days I could barely walk, and the pain kept moving about, through groin, quadriceps, calves, kneecap. X-rays of the lumbar area showed no serious vertebral damage, and no one, least of all myself, wanted to consider surgery. So I've been in physical therapy, trying to strengthen the muscles. Sustaining a back injury, the plague of caregiving, is a bit like being in an automobile accident. One second of carelessness and it takes months to repair the damage—*if* it can be repaired.

As I enter my bathroom, I become aware of my image approaching in the mirror. It is not a pretty or encouraging sight. I brace my hands against the porcelain basin and lean forward, peering into eyes where I can only imagine depth. Even without my glasses, which I left on the bedside table, I can see thin red lines running through the gelatinous whites of my eyes and disappearing into faded blue pupils. For a moment I feel a correspondence between the flatness of my image and my own being.

Kee not only bought furniture; she loved mirrors—round, rectangular, pentagonal, hexagonal, ornate and plain, framed and unframed. She even bought several known as "bull's eye." The name's well suited to a mirror which punctures self-preening as sharply as a portrait by Picasso, himself so adept at preening. But who am I to point fingers?

In other rooms mirrors reflect mirrors. Kee used to say that mirrors expand a room, but I suspect she liked them because they reflect movement and give some confirmation of reality. The mirror before me hangs over a massive porcelain sink. Like myself, it has seen better days. Some of the gilded plaster has chipped off, and some of its silvering is marred. It's not so imperfect as to distort, but it does underline blemishes. However, it's good enough for shaving, when I do shave, and it somehow abets the kind of wayward, inchoate ruminations which plague me much of the time.

I watch my hand, marked with liver spots and bulging veins, rub across gray stubble. Momentarily I am amused by the thought that I can make the hand disappear. I drop it to my side and the imaged hand disappears. I am the master of my image.

Perhaps I should shave. The imaged hand will mock me, but my hand will draw the blade. Then, thinking of the rich, white lather stained by flecks of gray swirling down the drain, I am repulsed, slightly frightened. I decide not to shave. And what if I never shave again? What if I let the stubble flourish, let it become long white strands, poetically blown by gentle breezes? Or perhaps it would become harsh, stringent, wirelike, exalting my image into a caricature of Old Testament prophecy? I like that thought. What shall I denounce?

Perhaps I fantasize like this because I am aging. My mind is as undisciplined as that of a four year old, jumping from one stimulus to another—willful, inconsistent. Yet I also know that the ordeal of Kee's Alzheimer's dementia has shaken whatever intellectual discipline I once possessed. The frequent irritability spawned by the necessity of confronting the minute-to-minute demands of living drives me toward thinking "what if. . . ."

With other people, friends and children, I think I usually seem to behave normally, listening to what is said, speaking coherently. Alone I am different. My mind darts about like a mouse in a maze, desperate, frenetic, as though activity alone might lead to escape. You think I exaggerate? Probably—a bit, but I'll give you an example of my inability to be at peace with myself. Over the last five years, I have gone to two movies alone. Both films were highly praised and the audiences seemed enthralled. In both instances I walked out before the movie was half over. I was simply unable to give myself to the experience, too many issues flooded my mind. I left the theaters and walked, walked with no objective, with no delight, and with no resolution of anything. I do not plan to go alone to films again.

I believe this heightened sense of critical self-awareness is common to the caregiver. Yes, note that I did not say a heightened self-understanding. Would that I could. Before the intrusion of AD into our lives, most choices, most actions seemed natural, simple. I lived within the text of life; now I feel relegated to the margin. I'm sure that other caregivers would explain this quite unpleasant state of being differently. I hope that some do not even feel the confusion I am trying to convey.

The image in the mirror seizes my attention again. Beneath the furry, disheveled eyebrows, I try to look through the windows of my soul. But I see nothing through the pane of glass. Verbalizing this fact, I frown at the pun—and wonder whether it's the pain in my soul that prevents my seeing anything. Do you like puns? Punning is a low form of humor. Maybe that's why I do it.

Mirrors fascinate me because they provide an audience. I need someone to talk to. I'd much prefer someone other than myself, but sometimes you have to make do, and frequently I'm starved for conversation. I don't say that lightly. My greatest loss is that of Kee as confidant and friend. I need someone to talk *with*, not just to. Someone else might keep my reflections honest.

Reflections: visual and nonvisual. To reflect could mean to think about something rather than to produce a reflection. To ruminate, as I have vaguely been doing, is only a thought process, yet it sounds heavy, ponderous, as though the only ideas upon which one can ruminate are in a junkyard full of rusting automobiles and old stoves. Memories, too, rust.

I take another look at myself/not myself, the predominant nose which, blessedly, has prevented my suffering the misfortune of being considered handsome, the oversized ears rising expectantly as if anticipating a distant voice, the large mole on my cheek, identifying me like a fingerprint. The white hair is thinning, the moles becoming darker. I stare at this face and mutter, "These are the golden years."

I think of my body's steady march toward dissolution and of the keening poem of decay in Ecclesiastes:

> In the day when the keepers of the house shall tremble,
> and the strong men shall bow themselves,
> and the grinders cease because they are few,
> and those that look out of the windows be darkened,
> and the doors shall be shut in the streets,
> and the sound of the grinding is low . . .
> when they shall be afraid of that which is high,
> and fears shall be in the way,
> and the almond tree shall flourish,

and the grasshopper shall be a burden,
and desire shall fail:
because man goeth to his long home,
and the mourners go about the streets:
Or ever the silver cord be loosed,
or the golden bowl be broken,
or the pitcher be broken at the fountain,
or the wheel broken at the cistern.
Then shall the dust return to the earth as it was:
and the spirit shall return unto God who gave it.
Vanity of vanities, saith the preacher;
all is vanity.

My unsteady hands, my bridges and titanium implants, my increasing deafness—all confirm the preacher's grim description. I've never quite figured out what is meant by the wheel broken at the cistern, but it sounds ominous enough. I do understand "desire shall fail." As for vanity or emptiness, I don't think my life has been entirely in vain. The preacher of Ecclesiastes professes to find nothing new under the sun, but I believe Kee and I found much that was new, new and sparkling with possibilities: one another, children, flowers, the earth and sea, the joy of other people, well, most other people. That it will all end in dust, dust and ashes, does not negate the beauty we have known and shared.

Bending toward the sink, I disappear from the mirror, splashing water on the face which, whatever its faults, is me—and I'm accustomed to it. It's the face I've earned, I suppose. Sometimes I even like it. I grope for the towel and dab at my face. Rehanging the towel on the edge of a shelf, I flick off the overhead light and limp through the door knowing that my darkening image will seem to exit through the same door and disappear.

Should I summon it back by turning? To what end? To resolve a falsely remembered past? All of the thousands of versions of my experiences—of people, places, things, and events are equally skewed, equally accurate, equally fictitious. Each memory is an act of creation. What is the point? To examine myself? Which self? To counterpoint past with present or even to examine being itself? Presumptuous! Absurd!

I do not turn to call the image back. Nor do I have any desire to wave a cheery good morning. What's likely to be cheery about it?

Kee is still asleep, her legs now extend almost to my edge of the bed. Four years ago she had three serious falls. On one occasion I went outside briefly with our grandson while she was resting in bed. When we returned about twenty minutes later, we found her lying on the floor of my study, conscious but unable to rise. She had forgotten my telling her that I would be gone a few minutes and had come looking for me. I picked her up and carried her back to bed. The following morning when I moved her, she cried out. Any movement caused her to wince. Her doctor and I agreed that a trip to the hospital for X-rays would be traumatic in itself. Since the treatment would be bed rest, I chose to forego the hospital trip. In about eight days, she was well enough to stand and walk with assistance, but I had to be careful. If I didn't hold her securely, she would slip away and fall.

About a week later, I took her to the bathroom before her afternoon nap and asked her to remain on the commode while I took towels to a nearby closet. "Now, please, don't try to get up by yourself," I begged. Before I even reached the closet, I heard the noise of a body striking a door and whirled to see her plunging down the hall out of control. Before I could reach her, she fell headfirst into a door jamb. Blood from a gash in her scalp spewed over her face and clothes and over the door. I used one of the towels I was carrying to apply pressure to the gash. Within several minutes the bleeding subsided.

Carefully, I thought, I gathered her up and returned her to bed. I cut away hair around the gash, cleaned the wound, and rubbed on Neosporin. Then I called her doctor. Unfortunately, it was a Sunday, and he was not on call. I talked with another doctor who advised me to take her to the emergency room. Not knowing Kee, he had little sense of how traumatic an emergency room and X-rays would be. Nor did he understand that an operation would be a last resort. Thus I found out the hard way that caregivers need to work out with their doctors how to cope with emergencies when their primary care physicians are not available.

By Monday it was clear that her back was damaged again, either from the fall or from my lifting her. I talked with her doctor this time. Again we agreed that the best course of action was to let her rest in bed, not getting her up even to go to the bathroom. A week or so later, however, she crawled out of bed and fell again. That's when I got bars for the sides of the bed. Soon it became evident that she could not put much weight on her left leg, and carrying her weight on my right hip with my right arm under her shoulder was forcing my spine out of line and inviting trouble. Already my back had begun to bother me. Moving her in a wheelchair was the only solution. Without it I would no longer be able to care for her.

Avoiding waking Kee, I check to make certain that she is still on the waterproof pad and run my hand softly across her forehead. She will probably sleep somewhat fitfully for another hour.

I pick up my glasses. Without them I can read nothing much smaller than a billboard. For forty-five years the skills of ophthalmologists and lens craftsmen have guided me through the progression from single lens to bifocals to trifocals. One pair I use only when golfing— a tinted pair with the reading lens placed in a small arc at the top of the glass so that the golf ball at my feet will remain relatively clear. With the small lens I can read a score card if I remember to lower my head in the manner of Ben Franklin peering suspiciously over the top of his glasses at his fellow delegates to the Continental Congress. For handball I use protective glasses that let me focus my eyes on a point about ten feet away. Wearing them, I can follow the course of the ball but can't read the numbers on the combination lock at the gym. The complex mechanics of sight, the marvels of technology, the miracles of my body, all things I usually take for granted until failures capture my attention.

My ophthalmologist recently announced that the first signs of macular degeneration are evident. Disgruntled by this further whisper of decay, I think what a limited portion of what I actually see registers. Why do my eyes transmit so much to the brain that I cannot recall? Or so much that is incidental or irrelevant—the thin layer of dust on the bedside table, the ash from my overturned pipe, an old grocery list? I understand only a little of the physics of sight and even

less about the perplexing phenomena of perception and understanding. But the intriguing word to me is *vision*. Is that a phenomenon we all share? A special gift? This speculation is quickly ended
with a self-deprecating snort. Vision is not a quality I possess. I am
pedestrian.

Mulling over the ingenuity of eye specialists, sour from my too early encounter with the mirror, I put the glasses on. By donning them
I acquiesce to whatever challenges the day may bring. As I start toward the kitchen, I pass my dresser, where I keep the picture of Kee
taken for the announcement of our engagement. She was beautiful
then. This picture helps me recall how she looked—the radiant smile,
the hint of dimples, the unfurrowed brow—before the ravages of
Alzheimer's. For years I kept the picture in my study but recently
moved it to where it acts as an antidote to the recent images acidly
etched in my mind—the uncomprehending gaze, the unresponsive
body.

In the kitchen I reach into the cabinet where I keep the cereal, then
remember that I finished a box the day before. Damn! Damn, damn,
dammit. For a moment I consider having half a grapefruit and a
piece of toast, but if I do, I'll be eating cookies before lunchtime, seeking the solace of sweets, yielding to the siren call of cream fillings. Besides, the unopened cereal will still confront me tomorrow, again testing courage and will. Reluctantly, I pull the box down and obediently
insert the thumb of my right hand where the instructions say OPEN
HERE. Pulling one flap away from the other is no problem. That's not
what frets me. What now faces me is the task of opening the sealed
plastic container, something I once did effortlessly, thoughtlessly.
Now the task is Herculean. I place the thumb and forefinger of my
right hand on one side and the thumb and forefinger of the left on
the other and pull. My left hand slips helplessly off, weakened by
shingles, by a pinched radial nerve, perhaps merely by muscular at-
rophy. Or is there some alien force—the old World War II use of
"gremlins" pops into mind. Angrily I grab the plastic again, hoping
the time will come when with both hands I can throttle the idiot vice
president of packaging who sends such trials into the world. Vengeance, I grunt—but fantasies don't open cereal packages.

I try again and fail again. The inability to accomplish so simple a
task infuriates me. I jerk open a drawer where scissors are buried under old knives, broken spatulas, and an egg timer, things I've never
bothered to throw away. As a boy I took to heart the motto "Be Pre-

pared" and now find that roughly equivalent to collecting junk. With the scissors I savagely jab a ragged hole in the plastic. In some vital whirl of the cortex there is a laugh. To laugh at my frailty, at my desire for revenge, to laugh because laughter is, perhaps, the only hope seems wise, but I can manage only a wry smile. I still regret that my hands are unstained with the blood of an anonymous vice president of a vast and profitable bulwark of the food industry—anonymous, but not innocent.

The cereal tumbles into the bowl, neither bowl nor cereal offering resistance to their coupling. There are strawberries in the refrigerator. Because the nerves of my left thumb no longer signal eminent danger, I slice them with exquisite care. Placing a coverlet of strawberries over the cereal, I reach into the refrigerator again, taking out a plastic jug marked MILK 1% FAT, and thoroughly douse my breakfast.

Only after pouring the milk do I realize that I forgot to prepare the automatic coffeemaker last night. Damn! Now I have to choose between eating crisp cereal and then waiting fifteen minutes for my coffee or fixing the coffee first, then eating soggy cereal. This is the second time this week that I've forgotten to prepare the coffee before going to bed.

Why have I unintentionally abandoned my rituals? How can I begin a day so distracted and confused that I can't even follow old habits? Alzheimer's disease! I am its victim. Then I recognize yet again that my rage is least governable when I am not with Kee. In some strange way, her presence is soothing. This awareness distresses me, and I make an effort to tamp down my bitterness.

I decide to eat the cereal while it is still crisp, so I pull up a stool by the kitchen counter and sit down—alone. Because I have not yet picked up the paper, I turn to the cereal box and for what seems the thousandth time read the nutrient list. I am promised 25 percent of my daily requirement of vitamin A, 25 percent of calcium, 25 percent of iron, and, intriguingly, the *same* percentage of thiamin, riboflavin, niacin, vitamin B, folic acid, phosphorous, and zinc. Why a quarter of my daily needs, not 30 or 60 percent, but always 25 percent (except for the tad of magnesium and copper thrown in almost like an afterthought)? How can I *know* that there are not 28 percent of folic acid requirements and only 19 percent of zinc? With keener interest I note that one serving contains three grams of fat, consisting of one gram of polyunsaturated fat, one gram of monounsaturated fat, and no saturated fat. That doesn't add up. How can a cereal company add one and one and get three? What's unaccounted for? What unnamed substance makes up that missing gram? I know the question is absurd, that I will never profit from this surfeit of nutritional information of dubious accuracy, but I keep reading.

According to the information provided, I am expected to consume sixty-five grams of fat daily in a two thousand calorie diet. I have no idea what my caloric intake is. Counting calories interferes with the pleasures of consumption. The secrets of a Snickers bar should be honored. Besides, according to Discovery the previous evening, bears know instinctively how much fat they need to pack on for hibernation. Why shouldn't I possess the same instincts even if I've never succumbed to the temptation to hibernate?

It occurs to me that bears in zoos do not hibernate, at least those in the zoos I have visited. How do bears know that their keepers will daily provide scientifically determined grams of fat? Can thousands of years of evolution be undone so quickly? How and why have animals so quickly adjusted to man's control? If a bear could talk, would he say to his keeper, "Please, kind sir, I need 500,000 calories today because I'm going to take a long nap?" Surrounded by moats and fences, brushing against concrete boulders, the sluggish captive adjusts meekly to his keeper's cycle of working and sleeping. In his dreams, does a bear mourn for his lost hereditary patterns, or does he gloat that food comes so regularly with so little effort?

Habit—when to wake, when to eat, when to work, when to eat again, when to sleep—momentous questions resolved by habit. I remember one of my uncles, a train dispatcher who worked the night shift. Holidays were a disaster for that uncle and his family because on vacation he was expected to observe a more normal schedule. One day of irritability followed another until the vacation ended and he contentedly returned to work and his accustomed schedule. Unlike my uncle, I'm now beginning to adjust habits that have served me well. Why am I altering them, and so unwittingly, even a habit so negligible as making coffee?

Shoving the cereal box away, I eat the final few spoonfuls of cereal and then begin to make the coffee. There are still no sounds from the bedroom. Having started the coffee brewing, I retrieve the newspapers from outside the front door.

Retirement has given me the leisure to read the morning papers slowly. Unfortunately the leisure has also made me a vassal of television news—the *NewsHour with Jim Lehrer, CNN Headline News,* local news. The expectancy my parents felt every morning as they opened their paper is a lost pleasure. News in the local paper has the quality of soggy cereal. The stories add little substance to the news of the previous evening—except for an occasional sports score. What I used to call the funny pages aren't. I can't remember when I last chuckled aloud over a "comic" strip.

Scanning the predictable headlines, I wonder at my ability to grant myself immunity from pain. People—human beings by the thousands—are dying in crashes, drowning in floods, being ripped asunder by explosions. Children with bloated bellies compete with pedophiles for my attention, and I am so accustomed to reported misery that I feel no pain. While sipping coffee I maintain an eerie distance from those who suffer, at least those who suffer physically.

I've never actually seen anyone starve nor have I seen bullet-torn bodies except through the images in papers, magazines, television, and film. Between newsreels and movies there is no visible distinction, no discernable difference between the real victims and the actors who rise from the carnage unscathed. In the end, neither delivers more than momentary distress.

Maybe providing vicarious experience is the principal function of the media, a vicarious experience which anesthetizes the viewer, providing such an excess of pain that by habit we become like battle-hardened veterans who learn to look the other way. Surely an anthropomorphically conceived divinity would have to develop equivalent insensitivity. Man can bear less pain than he thinks. How does one survive but by not knowing, or, if one must know, by not feeling? I have cause to know that my tolerance for pain is limited.

After scanning the front page to refresh my memory of what is, for the nonce, newsworthy, I open the paper to page upon page of advertising: stores, automobile dealers, grocery stores, and building contractors among others—carnivores and herbivores all—foraging for survival.

The full frontal assault of advertisers clamoring for name recognition, touting their superiority, annoys me. I propose an absurd question: "What if all advertisers canceled their advertising and used their savings to reduce prices?" Such speculation gives me an odd satisfaction. I create dialogues with myself, haranguing a one-person audience, offering rebuttals. Knowing full well their absurdity, I follow random thoughts like a yellow brick road, hopeful of finding some wizard at the end. I told you I'm crabby.

Think of a world free of advertising executives, a world where television programs, few in number, would be automatically charged to the viewer through some mechanical device. Prices of magazines would soar, and that in itself would blessedly reduce their number. Forests would be saved. Billboards would disappear from the landscape. Quality of product and quality of service alone would count.

Internal laughter reminds me that the whole bloody economy would collapse. Millions would be laid off, plants would close, corporations would go bankrupt; my own savings, all paper, would be consumed as in a fiery furnace with no angels. Catastrophe! And all for the want of advertising, the nail that holds the horseshoes on the steeds of kings of capitalism. I say to myself what Kee would once have said: "You're being silly."

You think so, too, I see. Yes, I tend to digress. Sorry, but you need to know something about the ways I react to normal day-to-day absurdities before you can understand how I deal with tragedy. The comic and the tragic are intertwined, don't you agree? Anyway, I'm getting to Kee's story—and mine. Be patient. If you can't be patient, you'll never make it as a caregiver.

As I shove the paper away, I notice that it is Saturday. Preoccupied with my irritability, unable to curb a grinding anger that can turn any object—the morning paper, a cereal box, a mirror—into enemy or impediment, I have not been aware that the weekend is here. For the next two and a half days, I will have no relief. On the weekends, I care for Kee alone. Weekends sometimes stretch into unfathomable reaches of time.

For the past two years, I have not left my wife alone in the apartment for more time than it takes me to empty the trash. If Kee thinks that she is alone, she becomes agitated. There is also the chance that she might try to climb over the bars of the bed and fall. For the next fifty-two hours, I will be on full-time duty. In one sense, I do not object and am even pleased that I can still perform this service. The cooking, the washing, and most other chores are not difficult.

What distresses me as I approach a weekend is the awareness of the solitude and loneliness I will feel. Kee is here but not here. I talk with her. She might smile, but she does not understand. She might even speak, but what she means can only be guessed at. And with myself I am grouchy, irritable—lousy company to be stuck with. Particularly on the weekends I want to return to a distant past, to recreate what we once shared, to explode the nightmare of my waking hours.

After pouring another cup of coffee, I begin counting our pills. We each take four, but they differ except for the vitamin pill apiece. The seven bottles on the table give the impression of a small pharmacy. Yet for some of our contemporaries four pills is a small number. I used to resent having to take medicine, but now pills are a standard part of our daily routine, a crutch I no longer resist.

Every morning for more than nine years I have dispensed Kee's medicine like a diligent druggist. Originally, we expected that the drugs would lead to some improvement, but they didn't help and instead probably added to her sluggishness. With her doctor's approval, we stopped using them. Now she takes only "maintenance" medication: synthroid, ritalin, tegratol, a multivitamin. I lay them out and she takes them faithfully, without complaint. Now, of course, I have to give them to her one at a time. My medications are two ibuprofen tablets for my leg pain, a Paxil for depression, and a multivitamin.

Pill taking is, I fear, essentially another habit, a way of slogging through another day, another week, until. . . . The word *until* quivers in my mind, seeking its object. Its use anticipates a change of horizons, something appearing over the ridge, like the cavalry in a Western when settlers are surrounded. The object of *until* has changed over the years. Initially it was *until she is better.* When hope for a miracle died, it became *until she dies,* but I cannot imagine a future where she is not present. More often, of late, it reads *until I die,* a very real possibility but equally incomprehensible.

Our children don't have the resources to care for Kee, so we confront a serious dilemma. In the early stages of her illness, we half-seriously talked of suicide together—of some simple gesture intended not to deny life, but to assert an individual right, even obligation, to control fate as best we could. As her illness advanced, she became incapable of posing the issue, much less coming to any conclusion. And

I am incapable of acting for her. To prepare a fatal concoction, to use a plastic bag, to pull a trigger, to wield a razor blade—No! On myself, perhaps, but never could I willingly take her life. *Until . . . ?*

If she were able to ask me, to beg that I help her die, I might have the strength to carry out her wishes. Now she is beyond making such a request. I will never know how I might have responded.

Sharing life I understand. For nearly fifty years we've shared one another. Thinking much alike, enjoying many of the same things, working toward similar, if vaguely conceived, objectives, bringing children into life and seeing them safely through to adulthood—sharing. But sharing death? I understand the words, the syntax, but not its implications.

There are days when death seems alluring, enticing, sexy—like an airbrushed pin-up. Like the pin-up, desire for death is entirely fantasy. My will to live is enfeebled, but it persists like an annoying wart. For the present, at least, suicide is not an option. The quality of my life has shriveled, but there are still too many things remaining to experience, perhaps to suffer. I no longer expect rapture. I've known joy, even rapture. But that's past tense. Now I am driven by one thing— she needs me.

Although most of Kee's time is spent in the mists beyond consciousness, in a curious way she is as present as she has ever been. She is less than a fully cognizant person but more than a mere body. And I do not know what I mean when I declare that.

From the bedroom I hear a weak cough, then another, slightly stronger. Kee is waking up, drowsy, perhaps, but awake and expecting me. Whether she needs to cough every morning when she wakes, I don't know. Because of her smoking, perhaps she does. In any event, her second cough has become my signal. Some mornings, if it is getting late, I go to the bedroom before hearing a cough to see if she is awake. Never. Only when I hear the second cough am I certain that I'm being summoned.

She is lying on her left side when I enter the bedroom. Propping herself up, she raises her head and smiles. No matter how miserable I feel, no matter what muscle aches or how badly I slept, the smile warms me as an open hearth would. Most mornings there is a smile. I make idle chat, wish her a good morning, and place a fresh disposable slip-on within easy reach, then get her a clean shirt or gown. Sometimes she complains that she is just lazy. It's like a game. I say, "No, you're not lazy." She may respond, "I just don't do anything."

If I say, "What would you like to do?" she has no response, so usually I say, "That's O.K., did you sleep well?" And she usually responds, "I think so."

I swivel her around so that legs and feet hang over the side of the bed. Often as I move her, she will say "Goodness gracious" or "Mercy me" but none of the phrases carry any real feeling or perception. Sometimes I resent the fact that she never asks me whether I've had a good night's sleep, but then I know I'm feeling sorry for myself. She knows I am here. I know that she wants me here, and she is responding to me. It's just that her mind cannot reach beyond the narrow limits of her own needs.

At night I have to place two extra pads in the slip-on to absorb the urine. They always make changing her more difficult, but with scissors I cut the elastic straps and tug away everything. Then I pull her to her feet briefly and rub baby oil or lotion on her bottom. Once I joshingly asked her if it frightened her to see me coming at her every morning with a pair of scissors. The question only confused her.

While she sits on the side of the bed, I pull a fresh T-shirt over her head and help her put her arms through the sleeves. T-shirts are easier for me to wash and more comfortable for her. Blouses or dresses are saved for those rare days when someone comes to see her. Rarely do I put a brassiere on her.

There is an art to putting on the slip-ons that took me a while to learn. For the first six weeks that I used them, Kee was confined to bed because of her falls. Any movement of her body caused pain, yet to get the slip-ons in position required lifting and twisting her. That's when I learned to use scissors to cut them away. I still had to move her to get clean ones on, but cutting them off gradually reduced the time she was in pain. Even now, because she can put weight on only one leg, I use the scissors. To put them on, I get her into a sitting position, put each foot, one at a time, through its leg hole, and pull the garment up as far as a sitting position allows. Then I bend my knees to protect my back, get her to wrap her arms around my neck, and then rise, bearing the weight almost entirely on my legs, telling her at the same time, "Now, stand up as best you can." Then holding her with one arm, I grasp the slip-on with my other hand and pull it into position. At first I had to feel for the slip-on with my free hand, but eventually I discovered that I could do the job more quickly if I used the full-length mirror on her closet door to see what I was doing.

Before placing her in the wheelchair, I embrace her fully, saying,

"Give me a hug!" The response physically is weak, but as always she says "Yes, yes." It is only 8:30, and the best of the day is over.

Once I get her settled into the wheelchair, I move it near her dresser, take a hairbrush and begin to brush out the tangles of the night. I've never really mastered this task, although one of the women who comes to stay with Kee has improved my technique. Kee winces whenever I draw the brush through her hair too forcefully. She doesn't complain, but sometimes there is an "ouch." The brush, one that allegedly produces less static, was picked out by my daughter. Once I get Kee's hair brushed back and relatively neat, through a series of clumsy maneuvers I work it into something approaching a ponytail and secure it with an elastic band. It's not elegantly done, but it keeps the hair out of her face. My daughter and the women who come on weekdays do her hair and nails with a grace and confidence I can't master. I'm almost certain that Kee prefers their doing everything related to personal toilet. Ten years ago she wouldn't have believed that I would even try to do things like brushing her teeth.

Once, years ago, Kee was down with the flu and feeling miserable. I thought I was doing a pretty good job of caring for her until she rose up on one elbow and declared, "I hope I never become seriously ill because you are a lousy nurse." That hurt. "Why, what did I do wrong?" I wanted to know. She glared at me, said, "Oh, forget it," and fell back on her pillow. Of course I haven't forgotten it, but I still don't know what her complaint was. Probably she was irritated by what I was not doing.

Now, I push the wheelchair into the dining room and up to the table, light Kee a cigarette and get her a cup of coffee. Her breakfast desires are modest. Although she used to eat cereal with me, for several years now she has refused it. I tried eggs, tried waffles, but found that the only thing she will eat for breakfast is pastry. That's easy enough. On Sunday mornings, in an effort to maintain some continuity with our old life, I prepare bacon and poached eggs on toast. With a little coaxing, she usually eats it all, but even then it's clear that she prefers her pastry. Blueberry is her favorite flavor. Why I insist on giving her some variety, I can't tell you. I suppose it's because I'm sure I would want variety. Sometimes I get cinnamon, raspberry, apple, or cherry. She eats them, but only blueberry brings pleasure to her eyes.

When Kee is eating she never says anything unless I ask, "Is it good?" Then she usually says, "I think so." I have to anticipate her readiness for each bite. If I offer it to her before she's ready, she will chew vigorously on some morsel tucked back in her cheek. If I wait too long, she reaches for a cigarette.

While she eats, I keep up a broken monologue: "It looks like it will be a nice day. . . . Last night's rain made everything fresh, but it also took more leaves down. . . . I don't think our grandson is coming today, but I'm sure he will tomorrow. . . . What would you like for supper tonight. . . . The paper says that they are still arguing about the extension of the light-rail system." Occasionally she answers with a nod or even a "Yes" or an "I don't know." Years have passed since she initiated any conversation. It seems longer. I'm not even sure she likes it when I talk to her. She seems content if I feed her, sit there with her, and light the occasional cigarette. I'm the one who needs the conversation.

When I rise to get her more coffee, I rub her neck or kiss her on the cheek. When I say, "I love you," she responds, "I love *you!*" but that declaration requires the prompt.

As I give her the morning pills the soiled deck of cards catches my eye. Another habit. I've reached for them before I even think about it. The cards are aged, the backs worn, the edges scarred. Early in Kee's dementia, I put a deck of cards on the table. Sometimes I sat with her for hours, playing hand after hand of solitaire. She wanted my presence, and because she grew troubled if I became engrossed in reading, I turned to solitaire. If she began a pattern of automatic speech, I could respond. Now she doesn't volunteer any speech except the occasional "maybe, maybe." I can shuffle the deck and play a hand quite automatically. If I miss an occasional move, it doesn't matter. The object is not to win but to keep occupied.

There is something satisfying about the simplicity of black seven to red eight, red jack to black queen, black three to red four, ace to the top row. The rules are neat and clear, choices few and of modest demand. Several years ago, when I became intrigued by probabilities, for three or four weeks I kept score of how many cards I "got up" and obsessively charted my success or failure, hand by hand, for two thousand hands. No. I'm serious. I played more than two thousand but didn't chart the rest.

Playing with numbers is as satisfying as playing the game—neither activity involves any stress on intelligence, and the results are utterly irrelevant to anything of value. I decided that those who keep baseball records (batting averages, earned run averages, stolen

bases, etc.) must have made the same discovery: that part of the pleasure of computation springs from the realization that such statistics
are utterly useless (except to a handful of millionaire owners and
players negotiating new contracts). So with solitaire. Although I become miffed when I think probability fails me for twenty hands in a
row, I also experience sheer delight, the sense of some heavenly blessing, when those same laws seem suspended in my favor and, against
all odds, turn up card after needed card. Once I won—really won,
honestly, no cheating—three times in eleven hands. I'm not enough
of a mathematician to calculate those odds, but for a few moments I
felt the rapture of being among the elect. I even began to understand
how a winning prize-fighter, after beating his foe senseless, might say,
"I owe it all to blessed Jesus, he done it all."

After keeping a record of two thousand games, I determined that
with even casual attention I am likely to win a hand—getting all the
cards into those four neat little piles—an average of one in twenty-
seven attempts. Although I've never seen solitaire played in a casi-
no, I'm told that when play is allowed, eleven up is a winning hand,
though not very profitable. According to my figures over two thousand hands, the average number of cards "up" is 8.35. The house
wins! The occasional victory will not threaten their coffers.

What intrigues me most, however, is that to beat the greatest odds,
you have to get skunked, to get no cards up at all! If you don't cheat,
getting no aces and, therefore, no cards up is ten times less likely
than turning up all the cards. Old Sol skunked me, gave me the to-
tal washout, only nine times in the two thousand hands—odds of
222.2 to 1. There must be a lesson in there somewhere, but I don't
think I want to know it.

The reason I've become fascinated with statistics may be my concern about whether our children might inherit a susceptibility to
Alzheimer's disease. I've read that a mutation on three separate chromosomes will cause the dementia, but that such anomalies account
for only 2 or 3 three percent of all cases. A gene possessed by many
people carries a susceptibility to Alzheimer-type dementia. Yet one
might have that susceptibility and never display any effects. What
are the odds that one or more of my children or my grandson will be
devastated by such dementia? Is Kee a carrier? Am I? One neurolo-
gist told me that he would strongly advise against genetic testing to
determine susceptibility, but he could not venture reassuring odds.
"We do not yet know enough," said the doctor. I'm sure he's right, but

sometimes I hear a nightmarish question pounding in my brain: "Are we all dangling on some prong of probability?" Yes, I like dumb alliteration, too. But really, what are the odds, and do I want to know them?

For now, I'm in no mood to play games of chance. I put the cards down but am still thinking about probability. What were the odds against Kee and I ever meeting? I knew her less than a week before I was certain that I wanted to marry her. What were the odds against my persuading her that she could and should "fall in love" with me? In June she declared that she did not plan to get married ever. By August, we were close to the question when we would marry. Looking back, we both felt that our romance was impetuous, and that we were unbelievably lucky. And we've defied the odds for over fifty years.

Kee was pretty, vibrant, intelligent, warm. More important, we shared so many values. By the standards of our place and time, we were considered "liberals"—against Jim Crow laws, opposed to nuclear proliferation, eager to contribute to what we perceived to be the improvement of the society. She wanted to work in counseling; I wanted to teach.

That summer she had a job as a waitress at a mountain resort. I arranged to visit her there, and we strolled mountain paths perfumed by late-blooming rhododendrons and mountain laurel. We sat by waterfalls and talked about what we wanted to do. As we courted, discovering one another's interests, moving toward engagement and marriage, the issues of offspring and genetic inheritance never crossed our minds. When I told her that I wanted to marry her, I think we both assumed that our lives would, like the setting, prove idyllic. Love was sufficient, or was it sexual attraction? It didn't matter. Only being together mattered. That her grandfather was afflicted with what was then called "hardening of the arteries" was also irrelevant. Love would sustain us.

Two years later, when she finished college, we were married. She would work while I completed graduate school. We moved north, where she found a position directing a young adult's program in a YWCA. We invested in two secondhand bicycles so that she could avoid the bus ride to work, and we could bike along the river for pleasure. Once we even made a forty-mile ride to the Y's summer camp near the ocean. Without question that was Kee's greatest athletic accomplishment.

Although some of the young women were older than Kee, they

came to adore her, confiding in her, inviting her to their private parties. Her colleagues praised her leadership and interpersonal skills. And I basked in the praise of this woman I loved.

Our lives expanded. We made friends, found a church we liked where the minister did not preach at his parishioners but guided us in a quest to understand spiritual dimensions. We walked to the grocery store together, trundling a wire cart between us. One night, after a movie, we came out into fresh snow and frolicked like the children we really were, tossing snowballs and making snow angels. We played bridge with other couples whose entertainment budgets were as strapped as our own.

When Kee returned from her first annual physical after taking her job, I knew the moment I saw her that she was troubled. She had been bothered by a cold. Could it be pneumonia? "What's wrong?" I asked. She dissolved into tears. She was pregnant, something we hadn't planned on. But how? According to the doctor, we simply hadn't been careful enough.

We comforted each other, reassured ourselves, and began to rework finances, trying to find some way that I could continue graduate school when she left work. We were both determined to welcome our firstborn and, in our youthful folly, to be ideal parents. I accepted a graduate assistantship, which took even more of my time, yet we convinced ourselves that everything would work out beautifully, and we had a handsome son to fondle and share. We found friends who passed along cribs and bassinets. Our parents sent money for a stroller, and we purchased a baby's seat for my bicycle so that we could continue our rides. We had a toy-making party, sewing bits of vinyl around foam rubber for soft blocks and making plywood cutouts of the Seven Dwarfs for the walls. Kee studied Ilg and Ames on child development and immersed herself in the practical suggestions of Dr. Spock.

Eight months after Paul was born, we discovered that we were again expecting. Not careful enough? Impossible! We had followed all the rules! The pregnancy continued, oblivious to laws of probability. Another son and Kee was living in a sea of diapers. Change, wash, dry, change, wash, dry—a cycle more relentless than that of the ancient, used washing machine we acquired. There was no dryer. If the day was clear, each diaper flapped gaily in the wind, but we did not share the gaiety. If the day was rainy, lines were strung throughout the bathroom and kitchen. Disposable diapers were unknown to us, and we couldn't afford a diaper service. A second bicycle seat enabled us to continue to ride, occasionally, but there was less joy and more frustration and pain in our daily lives.

I took a summer job as a milkman. So that I could get to the loading dock at the plant, we bought a prewar Pontiac for two hundred dollars. The odometer showed 45,000 miles. Whether that meant 145,000 or 245,000 or more, we never knew, but it ran. Near the end of the summer and the twelve-hour days, a customer approached me about living in his summer house near the beach. Kee and I talked the issue over carefully. With no rent to pay, we might just be able to remain solvent. The problem was that the house was thirty miles away from the university, We kept the car so that I could make the one-hour commute to school. And now we could take our sons out in inclement weather. Grocery shopping became easier.

What we failed to take into account was how isolated Kee would be or how my long hours spent at school and commuting would reduce the time I could help her. Two more pregnancies followed, both ending in miscarriage. The miscarriages left us empty and anxious. We no longer thought of life as idyllic, but we were together, we had two lovely boys, and that was almost enough. We managed.

Only years later did we discover the extent to which each of us had deceived the other during those years. Kee was lonely, depressed, exhausted, but could not share that with me lest I be distracted from completing my studies. I was either too preoccupied or lacked the sensitivity to recognize her suffering. Nor could I tell her that financial concerns and anxiety sometimes reduced me to tears. We sought to be cheery and optimistic in one another's presence. Protecting the other was the constant in our relationship. Still in our mid-twenties, we thought of ourselves as models of maturity. Beneath our masks we trembled with adolescent anguish.

Looking back on those years, and the subsequent birth of our daughter, I am amazed by Kee's stamina and endurance. At the time, I thought I was doing all I could to help—but a few loads of laundry here and there, a few dishes washed, the occasional preparation of a meal were as nothing to the responsibility she bore. Looking at her now, frail and wrinkled at only seventy-two, I wonder how much can be attributed to Alzheimer's and how much to the anxiety and stress of those early years of our marriage.

When our daughter started school, the boys were ten and eleven. Kee decided that it was time to return to work. She had been active in the P.T.A., Sunday school teaching, and civic organizations, but volunteerism did not satisfy her. She felt that the children did not require all of her attention and began to look for challenges. She found one. Although she had never had administrative experience nor worked with small children besides her own, she was quickly hired to run a preschool center associated with Head Start in a housing project. She was delighted, but some of our friends and neighbors were appalled. It's not safe; you'll be going through the projects in the dark; think what could happen to you, they said. Kee was unafraid.

Her affectionate nature and consideration won over not only the children but also their parents. At afternoon nap time, she usually rocked one of the children to sleep, a privilege so prized that she had to follow a fixed rotation scheme. She held them when they fell down, read to them, loved them. Some were so deprived, so emotionally undeveloped, that they clung to her, except when they were angry and tried to kick her. One four-year-old boy, sitting with her in the play yard one day, his arm across her lap, said, "When I get older I'm going to be white like you." Kee said, "No, Darrell, you have beautiful brown skin and you should be proud of it." The little boy looked at her arms—it was July—and said, "Well, you're getting darker."

I sometimes visited her at the center and watched her. She taught one very bright little boy how to read; she consoled a little girl whose father was taken off to prison; she worked with all the children to teach them self-respect. Walking through that allegedly dangerous project, she was frequently greeted warmly by adults who knew who she was, why she was there, and how she loved and respected the children.

Kee left the position only because I received a fellowship to work abroad. When we returned she decided it was time for her to obtain further training. I hoped she would choose a field that would lend itself to teaching so that our schedules would coincide. I also hoped, and expressed the hope, that she would wait a year or two until our indebtedness was cleared. We had argued before, of course, mostly about trivial things, but this became the most divisive argument of our marriage. She accused me of not wanting her to work because it would interfere with my own comfort and schedule. She was probably correct, but I argued that we didn't have the money to pay for graduate training.

At the time, none of the argument was amusing. The issue was resolved, not with words, but by her applying for and receiving a fellowship. What could I say? The only reasonable response was "Good for you. I'll help around the house as much as I can." I cooked dinner several times a week, did much of the laundry, and tried to be home when the children came in from school.

When it came to her graduate work, however, she did not want assistance. Oh, I helped type a few papers and did some proofreading for her, but she refused any assistance that might compromise her control of her own work. I found that I could help best by reading bedtime stories to the children and taking them to the park on weekends. In two years, she earned her master's degree in clinical social work with honors. Our children were as proud of her as I was.

When she graduated, she took a job in the youth center of the state hospital, a place that proved more dangerous than the projects. One evening when she came home I immediately saw red welts on her neck. A fourteen-year-old girl, known for violent rages, five inches taller and sixty pounds heavier than Kee, had become angry when Kee told her that she was not ready for a weekend pass. The girl seized her by the throat and threw her against a wall. Another staff worker saw what was happening and ran for a security guard. By the time the guard and staff member arrived, the girl was slumped on the floor sobbing, and Kee was kneeling by her, an arm around her shoulders, comforting her. Before going into private practice, Kee also worked in the psychiatric unit of a private hospital, where she trained medical students. They were somewhat less dangerous.

Through all of her work, Kee managed to keep our children at the forefront of her concerns. Now our children are again a major concern. I can commit myself to keeping Kee secure and comfortable during her long illness, but there is nothing I can do about their genetic inheritance. I can't even know whether they bear a double whammy of the gene that heightens susceptibility to Alzheimer-type dementia. I know that worrying is of no use, but how can I not worry? Chance, probability, will reveal itself in its own time.

Whatever occurs, I am convinced they were damned lucky to have a mother who loved them so tenaciously without suffocating them. If we have given them genes which are susceptible to dementia, we have also given them a foundation of love.

Kee finishes her coffee and is ready for another cigarette. I light one for her, hoping that she will smoke it quickly. I need to go to the bathroom. While she smokes, I put away the dishes, checking on her every minute or two.

You've been very polite, but I've noticed that you seem to disapprove of my letting Kee smoke. And I gather you also have some reservations about my giving her Scotch. No, I don't think it none of your business. Smoking is both a dangerous and a dirty habit. But think of it this way—how much harm can it do her now? Shortly after Kee was diagnosed, I talked with her internist and asked him the same questions you have on your mind. Should I let her have a drink at night? He responded, "Does she enjoy it?" I said she did, and his surprising reply was "Let her have as much as you can stand." Taken aback initially, I quickly realized that I can't stand to let her drink much. Her limbs become even weaker and she gets more confused unless I strictly limit the drinking. I do. As for the smoking, the doctor indicated that he wished we both had quit long ago, but that now I had to decide whether I wanted to try to drag her life out as long as possible or give her as much pleasure as possible in whatever time she has to live. That stated the issue clearly and made the decision easy. I'm not asking for your approval. I'm just indicating why I've done what I have and why I'll continue to allow her those few pleasures.

Kee has finished her cigarette. I pour her more coffee, tell her that I need to go to the bathroom and put the wash in. In the bedroom I gather up two sheets and three towels, enough for a wash, put them in a plastic bucket (they're wet), and limp back down the hall to my bathroom. Habit is the only explanation for my continuing to use the sink and commode just off my study. When we first moved to our apartment, the bathroom off the main bedroom became Kee's. If we were getting ready to go somewhere together, it was more convenient for us to use different sinks and toilets. Later, when she could not go out with me, I continued to use "mine." No, there are no designating signs on either door.

"My" bathroom is small but comfortable. Where the tub once was, the air-conditioning unit is housed. Also crowded into the small, windowless space is the stacked washer/dryer, an essential component of the caregiver's living space. I could do without air-conditioning and refrigeration, maybe without microwave or stove, but deprive me of running water and my washer/dryer and I wouldn't last a week. Six loads in one day is my record, I think, but twenty plus a week is common. The first load of the day goes in with soap and scented softener. I'll have the sound of swish/slosh to entertain me while I use the bathroom.

Only one other object of consequence is here—the magazine rack. Magazines, books, and crossword puzzles are stored there. I am convinced that such materials, handy to the potty (john, toilet, commode, or what you will), are a requirement of sanity. This cluttered but functional room is my retreat. If, as sometimes happens at Christmas, the apartment is too crowded with people, I retreat into this satisfying chamber. One of my sons once told me, "Dad, you are the poopingest man I know." While I don't bask in this superlative, I am grateful he did not select a more graphic verb.

When I approached my seventieth birthday, a friend asked me how I was planning to celebrate it. "Quietly," I said. "At my age a birthday is like a bowel movement—necessary, sometimes quite satisfying, but not something one needs to celebrate publicly." That I said such a thing implies that I thought it clever. That I remember it suggests much more.

I can't remember my potty training, but I suspect it was strict. My mother told me that she put woolen mittens on my hands to keep me from sucking my thumb. Although she never described how she housebroke me, I observed with interest her training of our dogs. She swatted them on the nose with a rolled newspaper. If she left psychic scars in my tender sensibility, I am oblivious to them. Nor do I remember what wool tastes like. My mother can rest in peace. I have no desire to blame her—although she may have played some unwitting part in the development of my still-adolescent humor.

I survived youth as a relatively happy child holding no grudges against my parents. My own experiences as a father convince me that one can only do the best one knows how and that whatever is done will be declared obsolete, perhaps even cruel, within a few decades.

Neither children nor parents change very much fundamentally, but theories of child training arise, flourish, and die with astonishing rapidity.

A *New York Times* crossword puzzle will keep me company during my stay in the bathroom. Yes, I like crossword puzzles and am relatively strict on myself when doing them. No dictionary, no thesaurus, no encyclopedia. If a biblical passage is used that I can't quite recall, I might look that up. And Shakespeare. Oh yes, once in a while an atlas, but nothing else. I justify consulting the Bible and Shakespeare because both are voluminous and the atlas because maps have been drawn and redrawn over and over since my boyhood. Names changed— cities, regions, countries—as colonial powers withdrew in the face of nationalist zeal. Maybe Kipling is to blame for the fact that I can rarely recall the currently correct name for Burma.

I have a relatively informed grasp of the size and shape of Africa, but once I get past the nations on the Mediterranean, I can't name or locate half the countries between there and South Africa. And how long will that country bear an English name? Where is Rhodesia? Long gone.

Crossword puzzles fascinate me. To decipher the code that the creator of the puzzle imposes on the squares is an adventure. But what really interests me is filling in the blanks. Nature is said to abhor a vacuum and so do I. I usually finish the puzzle in an in-flight magazine before we leave the runway. On the other hand I've kept *New York Times* puzzles around for weeks without ever finishing them. I prefer to do a puzzle number by number but usually have to resort to flanking maneuvers. Decipher the code, discover the secrets, understand the pattern, fill the blanks, complete the puzzle, symbolically defeat ignorance yet again. Control! Compulsive and anal? Who, me?

The puzzle I'm working on now is one I started last night. It's a "step quote." The tricky aspect of such a puzzle is the absence of solid spaces in the quotation. Confronting forty-three consecutive open spaces, which turn downward and sideward rather whimsically, having no clue to the length of any of the words, I find the challenge formidable. Solving the step quote requires the "flanking maneuver," filling in intersecting answers you hope are accurate. Last night I filled in about half the spaces, yet still have no clue to the quotation's content, nor am I certain of a single word in the quotation.

I ignore the quotation and concentrate on its author. If I come up with a ten-letter word suited to "item that gives confidence," I'll get the clue I need to guess the author's identity. If I had a "search and find" key for my brain, this would be a snap. A seven-letter word for "forceful" at last pops up—*dynamic*. With dynamic I can fill in *Ibn* ("___ Saud") and *Turin* ("city on the Po") and then figure out that the answer to "item that gives confidence" is *credential*. The creator of the puzzle and I disagree on the appropriateness of that definition, but it's his puzzle. Anyway, with all of that in place I work out that the author of the step quote is George Santayana. Now who in hell would choose a quotation from Santayana for a step quote. No help at all.

Eventually, some fifteen minutes later (I've got to get back to Kee), I work out the quotation: "Life is not a spectacle or a feast. It is a predicament." My greatest difficulty was in working out "predicament." Fitting! Thank you Mr. Santayana for that rather trite observation.

But . . . I've succeeded. The puzzle is solved (or so I hope)—all the spaces filled. Victory! Patience, perseverance, imagination, the prescription for every aspect of life. I hustle back to the dining room carrying the book of puzzles with me. After chatting with Kee a bit and lighting a cigarette for her, I turn to the back of the volume of puzzles (remember, I don't "peek") to check results. Three errors! Egad! (By the way, are you old enough to remember Major Hoople? Ah well.) One error involves a city in California I have never heard of; another, a Greek port which intersects with a French king (Clovis?); and the third, an oversight where I forgot to change a letter when I changed my answer. A loser again. Add the cultivation of humility to the prescription for every aspect of life.

The telephone rings. As though wired to the phone, I jump, shocked out of my reverie. The suddenness of the movement is in contrast to my usual awkward, bone-weary rising from a chair, but the jangle of the machine is an intrusion I want to stop—now!

The phone rings a second time, more imperiously. As I stumble toward it, I strike my thigh against the edge of the buffet and swear. Even the furniture has turned hostile. I limp on toward the phone, determined to intercept the call before the mysterious wiring of the answering machine asserts itself. I dislike listening to the answering machine, and I'm afraid its tape will wear out and require replacing. I don't mind spending a few dollars on a new tape, but the inconvenience of finding a store that carries the correct tape (the machine is an old model) is a nuisance.

Then, too, there's the heritage I carry with me: "Waste not, want not." My mother, weaned on aphorisms, laid them on me. She inherited them from her father. I've managed to forget the phrasing of most of them, but the hard nut of their intent lies in the pit of my stomach, particularly those related to saving. In the kitchen are plastic bags and old aluminum foil, washed, dried, smoothed out, folded, ready for later use. "A penny saved is a penny earned." I collect rubber bands and scraps of wood from old projects. Once in a rare while I actually use something that I had tucked away in a nook or cranny, but using it is not the object. Saving is all. Why wear out a tape?

My collections are essentially of useless things. I uniformly failed to keep things that later came to have commercial value. The *Superman, Batman,* and *Captain Marvel* comic books of my boyhood were trashed before I entered high school.

Even my collection of baseball players' autographs, the only truly enterprising effort of my childhood, is gone, given to an ungrateful cousin. When about ten, I wrote short notes to my baseball heros, asking for their autographs on enclosed penny postals. In childish confidence I wrote only the name of the player, the team, and its far-off city on each envelope, expecting the U.S. Postal Service to take care of the rest. Stealing three-cent stamps from my father's desk, I confidently mailed the requests. Most of the letters must have reached their destinations, for the enclosed penny postal cards were usually returned. Over five years I amassed autographs of some of the greats and not so greats: Charley Gehringer, Hank Greenberg, Joe DiMaggio, Carl Hubbell, Mel Ott, Dick Bartell, Pinky Mahaffey. No one remembers Pinky now, but he once pitched for the Philadelphia Athletics when there was such a team. I liked his name. The one card I did not give to my cousin was from Lou Gehrig who had written "Best Wishes Burt, Lou Gehrig." I cherished the card and wept when Gehrig died with ALS. Since then I've lost two friends to the horrifying disease which bears his name.

There's one collection I've not thrown or given away. Throughout our many moves together, Kee and I have retained the love letters we shared in the two years before we were married. Safely tucked away in two cardboard boxes in the basement, marked His and Hers like bathroom towels, the letters haven't been read since they were put away more than fifty years ago. They are a bit like an insurance policy—not to be used but good to have. Perhaps our grandson will glance at them some day, seeing them as museum pieces, signs of an age long out of fashion. If so, he will have difficulty believing the current of passion surging through them. They will seem terribly dated, of course, quaint even, but although the language lacks the explicitness of current sexual language, any reader will detect the ardor. I suspect I might be a bit embarrassed reading them after half a century. I feel my ears take on a faint pinkish glow.

I get to the phone and snatch it up. To my gruff hello there is a moment of silence, then a click, then a recorded voice advising me that I have been selected to receive a valuable prize—a prize already in escrow for me. To receive full information about my good fortune, I should remain on the line. I want to do something violent, but I know the machine on the other end will register no difference between a violent breaking of the connection and a gentle one.

Before Kee lost all connection with reality, she was an easy victim of such calls. Magazine subscriptions flowed in. Tickets for alleged charity events appeared with demands for payment. We suddenly became "owners" of lots in new vacation developments. Siding companies appeared at the door of our condo eager to begin work until reminded that attaching siding to a tenth-floor apartment would be no easy task. Our long distance service was changed three times, each time without written confirmation, each time without any effort to verify.

How many telephone sales do you guess are made to similar victims, to persons who, because of age or illness, can understand neither what the call means nor the consequences of the response they make?

Several times I was at home when Kee answered sales calls. I heard her answer pleasantly, wait a few minutes, and then say, "yes," giving no evidence to the caller that she was unable to comprehend or act responsibly. The first time I heard her, she was well into reciting our address before I realized what was happening. Happily, even that early in the progression of AD, she had difficulty with numbers and could not give out credit card numbers.

For almost eighteen months after the diagnosis of Alzheimer-type dementia was first made, I continued to work, confident that she was safe at home alone for three or four hours at a time. Around noon I came home to check on her and prepare her lunch; otherwise she would have forgotten to eat. I was fortunate in that, unlike many of the disease's victims, she did not wander. Passivity was her normal behavior. Rarely did she express a preference; never did she show any inclination to go out. She responded to some stimuli, like the telephone, but otherwise lived in a distant world. At times we would have conversations in which she spoke alertly and seemed to understand fully what we were discussing. Then suddenly the conversation would derail, leaving us both bewildered. As the months passed, her speech became less coherent and more voluble.

During evening hours particularly, she chattered continually. Her words were easily understood but had no context or relevancy. One doctor called it "automatic speech." Words poured out, flowing on after the brain had lost its control system. She might sit at the table for an hour repeating phrases that were automatic: "That's O.K. isn't it . . . maybe, maybe . . . what do you think, maybe, maybe . . . I dunno, but maybe, maybe . . . but that's O.K. I think . . . do you reckon . . . I reckon . . . I reckon," which, of course, she could not do.

Unless I responded, the voice would continue like that on a cracked record, repeating over and over and over. Often I was torn between exasperation and the wish to respond to her. But to say something like "What are you asking?" led to confusion or produced "Whatever." In time I developed a shorthand of my own. If she said, "I just don't know," I learned to respond, "That's O.K., you know all you need to know," by which I meant, initially, that she had all she absolutely needed—a place to live, food, clothing, and one who would take care of her and love her. As months, then years, dragged past, I realized that my response was becoming less charged with meaning. It was tired, like myself. Was the comment merely a way of distracting her? I can't be sure.

Over the last two years the automatic speech has given way to silence. If I speak to her with the proper inflection, she will respond, but the response is to my tone, not my words. If I laugh at something, she might join me. If I comment angrily on something political, her body stiffens as though the anger were directed at her. I then must soothe her, less with words than with touch—holding her hand gently or caressing her shoulders.

One of the many things Kee taught me is that communication is more than words. When we were first married, she pointed out how little the members of my family touched one another. She was right. I recall being held as a child by both parents, but as we all aged, the laying on of hands was rare. My brother and I rarely touched one another, except in anger. It was as though each of us lived in a fragile glass bubble that might shatter if touched. Kee taught me the importance of touch—not only with her but also with our children and our friends.

Many years ago one of my friends was hospitalized for manic depression. I visited him in the hospital several times. When he was better, and given short passes, I brought him home one sunny afternoon to sit with us on our patio. Kee was gracious, as usual. I was pretending, more or less, that everything was "normal," that this was just an ordinary afternoon visit. At one point, Kee got up from the table, went over to him, and began to massage his neck and shoulders. That would never have occurred to me. My friend has never forgotten that act of affection and concern. Where words fail, hands and the warmth of the body speak forcefully. When my sons leave after a visit home to return to their own cities, their own duties, the profound communication lies in the parting embrace, not in the words.

Long after I became painfully aware of how little Kee's brain could process, my own need to communicate led me to comment on stories in newspapers and magazines, to describe my afternoon on the golf course, to tell about the activities of friends. The act of telling was more important than whether she did or did not understand. Sometimes she looked at me as if she understood. If I posed a question, frequently she would smile and say "maybe, maybe." More frequently of late, her chin is lowered nearly to her breast as though she is lost in thought. Again and again I wonder: "What does go on in her mind?" She cannot say. I cannot guess.

The absence of any genuine exchange gives me a dreadful sense of isolation. Part of her, an important, essential part, simply isn't there. She has a voice, which is the same as it has always been. She sometimes smiles with the warmth and graciousness that characterized her before she was afflicted. When we get to a doctor's office and the nurse welcomes her, Kee will smile broadly and say "Hello, hello!" I wonder sometimes if nurses think I exaggerate her condition. Once we were visited by old friends whom we had not seen in years. For the first ten minutes, her social ease was so effective that she seemed to them the woman they had known years before.

On occasion her brow will furrow and she will say, "Something's wrong, I think," but I never know whether she understands that something is indeed wrong or whether the phrase means anything specific to her. I've come to recognize that sometimes the phrase means she wants a cigarette and can't locate one, even if it is at her elbow. Or it might mean she doesn't want the rest of the food on her plate, or it might be that she wants something to drink.

For a while I read about communication problems for Alzheimer's victims—agnosia, anomia, aphasia, apraxia. The more I read, the more I sensed that the terms were useful to researchers but useless to the caregiver. It doesn't much matter whether the problem is with the victims' lack of recognition of persons or objects, or with substitution of nonsensical words, or with the inability to call up words once part of their vocabulary, or with translating thought into action. Living with Kee's confusion and meeting her needs are not resolved by categories. Even if I could identify the precise nature of her communication difficulties, that discovery would have no utility. It would only give me the illusion of understanding.

Distracted by these thoughts, I remain holding the receiver. Now a voice speaks: "Good morning, we are so pleased that you are accepting our valuable offer." Here is actually a human being on whom I can vent my anger, denounce for taking advantage of persons suffering from dementia. Then I picture a woman so in need of income that she is reduced to telephone solicitation. The profits of whatever scheme is being sprung will never go to her. I quietly hang up, denied even the satisfaction of rage.

When I return to the dining table, Kee does not even look up. There is no question like "Who was that?" or "What was that about?" I compress all that has gone on in the last few minutes into one sentence: "It was a solicitation call." For a brief moment, I wryly consider to whom I might place a solicitation call, but even "Ma" Bell has gone away.

The telephone's insistent ring destroyed the silence. As we sit together at the table in the mornings, I sometimes have the sense that I am being bathed gently by silence. Our apartment is on the tenth floor. Because the windows are thermal, not even the sound of trucks or automobiles from the street below reaches us. Occasionally the harsh, throbbing beat of a traffic helicopter or the wail of a siren intrudes, but normally silence prevails, a silence that I cherish—sometimes.

Silence is a strange phenomenon, isn't it? It can bring inner stillness, even joy. It can also intimidate to the point where I want to scream just to break its bonds. For me, I think the difference lies in whether I have a perception of sharing or one of acute loneliness.

The absence of intrusive sound this morning reminds me of our vacations in Colorado where we own a few acres, a bunkhouse, and several tents. We haven't been there now in six years and may never go again. Could I stand being there without Kee?

At nine thousand feet, isolated from the incessant demands of our work, we found solitude, not loneliness: the satisfying sense of being alone together and in harmony. Birdcalls blended into the setting unobtrusively—even if it was the harsh cry of a western jay or a Clark's nutcracker. Chipmunks raced about noiselessly or sat observing us, the intruders, from rock outcroppings. The occasional Golden Eagle or Red-Shouldered Hawk circled silently above us. Hummingbirds darted about, the whirr of their wings accentuating the silence. A jetliner might pass, leaving its trail in the sky, but at so high an altitude we would not hear it. Such silence had a creative, healing element to it. Silence, solitude—but that of our own choice.

Why does silence sometimes intimidate? I haven't quite worked that out. It's not entirely a matter of being physically alone, but it is related to some condition of not sharing. The sharing may be with a person or with a landscape or a crowd. But persons, landscapes, and crowds can also frighten and turn the solitude into something approaching terror. So it's more, or less, than that.

This morning I sit with Kee peacefully, sharing time and place with her. Yet at other times, when we are also sharing time and place in silence, I feel the terrifying loneliness. Maybe it depends on orientation, on whether I feel I have a sense of direction.

I once described to a friend the experience of living with AD by saying that it's like being dropped into the Everglades on a cloudy night without flashlight or compass. The darkness smothers and the imagination breeds terror. You know you must keep moving but have no idea which direction is least dangerous. I know that sounds overly dramatic. Perhaps I concocted it as a plea for pity—pity that I would have resented had it been offered. In fact I've never succeeded in measuring the dosage of pity I need, but it's an unwanted addiction. My craving for pity is fully matched by my resentment of it.

Being stranded, feeling alone, is not the same thing as solitude, which I think of as a sense of joy in separateness, of fully recognizing that one is alone, even reveling in the certainty of being alone, but at the same time not *feeling* alone. I knew such solitude often with Kee, but rarely in the presence of others. More frequently I've known this positive solitude when I was by myself—on a shore when a storm whipped the surf to frenzy or in the mountains when consciousness of seeing dissolved because I was enfolded in beauty. I've also known that joy of solitude in a cathedral when the organ completed a coda which seemed to drift slowly into eternity. In such solitude the prevailing sense is one of awe, a breathless adoration before being, a profound contentment with is-ness. Sadly, such moments are all too rare—but I've at least experienced them. And I am thankful that Kee and I have known them together, but that was before Alzheimer's intruded with shattering force.

This morning just being in Kee's presence is satisfying. At other times I feel all too acutely the isolation and loneliness because she is present but not present. Then the silence terrifies, producing panic. I first knew that silence when, at thirty-nine, she was diagnosed as having renal carcinoma, and I sat paralyzed by her bed in the hospital. Although the diagnosis was reversed a few days later, I won't forget that time. There must have been normal hospital sounds around me, but I heard nothing but the throbbing of my own heart and felt nothing but my own silent agony. How could I manage without her? How could I ever give the children what she gave them?

During Kee's long ordeal with Alzheimer's disease I have had a similar feeling arising not from the potential of her loss but from its present reality. Let me relate a particular incident that may help explain what I mean.

I woke up one morning with pain in my left arm and began to fear heart trouble although I've had no serious heart anomalies. I called my doctor's office, described my symptoms, and was given an appointment for the next day. The following morning, as I bathed before going to the appointment, I discovered a few red blotches on my left arm. The doctor took one look and said "Shingles." I had heard about shingles but thought of the ailment as something that afflicted only people with serious neuroses and stupidly considered myself immune. The doctor explained that reaction to herpes zoster, the same virus that causes chicken pox, may be stress related.

By nightfall my elbow and wrist were throbbing. By the following morning my left arm was covered with blisters. The pain moved into my hand and shoulder. The pain was so intense that I could not sleep even with sleeping pills. My elbow and wrist felt like they were imploding. The medication given for the herpes seemed to have no effect, nor did it for the three weeks I was allowed to take it. For the first time in my life I asked for stronger pain killers and sleeping pills. In addition I swallowed handfuls of ibuprofen and still hurt. In spite of physical therapy and continuing medication, the pain continued. For more than five months I was submitted to MRI's and electronic testing of nerves. By the third month I was desperate. I wanted help of any kind from any source. My doctor asked me if I felt depressed. The question struck me as stupid. Of course I was depressed. Couldn't he see that? Then I realized that it was the first time I had ever admitted to myself that I was genuinely depressed, not just having a bad day. I began taking an antidepressant that same day.

One evening, following supper, Kee and I settled down before the television. At that time she could walk and, even if she didn't watch the screen, at least sat with me. I have no idea what we were watching. I only remember that I began to cry—not for a fictitious character in a melodrama, not for Kee, but for myself. The neat world I had constructed was splintering. Financial plans made on the assumption of my continuing good health now seemed folly, and, above all, I was hurting. I tried to tell Kee of my pain and fears. She could not understand. Against every intention, I found myself sobbing, "If I can't maintain my health, I'll have to place you in a nursing home."

I had never, never meant to threaten her. To my surprise she was not disturbed. What I said was meaningless to her. Nor could she remember that I was hurting. If I said, "My wrist feels like there's a bonfire in it," she would respond sweetly, "I'm sorry," and mean it, but within minutes she would have no recollection either of my pain or her response.

The following morning after a fitful night half spent roaming the apartment, I was still immersed in pain and bedeviled by fears. Thinking her more lucid in the early morning, I tried yet again to communicate. "Do you understand why I was crying last night?" Pausing for a moment as if trying to recall, she said quite simply and accurately, "No, I don't." I cried again, my body shaking with frustration and hopelessness.

That is the terrifying silence of Alzheimer's—a silence arising from the noise of voices not communicating. It produces a sense of utter isolation because the person present, one with whom for years sharing was the essential fabric of life, is simply not there.

We experienced so many productive silences together. I was always the one given to chatter, as though fearful of the still moment. She was quieter, more aware of the communication that can occur in stillness. Fifteen years before the diagnosis of her dementia, we moved into a large home with an outdoor patio in a quiet section of the city. Except in winter, we ate our evening meal on the patio, lingering there over coffee or wine until well into the darkness, sharing the events of our days sometimes, but often allowing the silence to work its own magic.

Enough light came from neighboring yards and distant street lamps to give all the illumination we needed, although sometimes we lit candles or an old-fashioned kerosene lantern for "atmosphere." One night, as the darkness deepened and we sat in pleasant silence, a neighbor turned on a garage light and I became aware of something not previously noticed, something new. Between the eaves of our back porch and the corner of the patio wall, a spider had spun an enormous web, a web perhaps as much as three feet in diameter. The light from the neighbor's garage converted it into a shimmering work of art. Without a word, I pointed to it and Kee turned to see. For some time, we were quiet until at last she said, "That is so beautiful." Then I began to babble about how large a spider was required to spin a web of such size, to speculate on the kind of spider, to wonder how long it could withstand wind and rain, to note that the design was adapted to the need of the spider to work between two surfaces. The moment of beauty lay in the silence between our first discovery of its existence and my rattling on about minutiae. The silence honored the beauty of this work of nature far more than my enthusiastic babble. But we both knew that the beauty was enhanced by our seeing it together.

There were also the campfires each summer when we took our children into national forests and later, with the children encumbered by the responsibilities of their own lives, when we camped on our land in Colorado. The fires were prepared during daylight hours, then lit as the sky darkened. For two or three hours we watched the progression of the fire as it blazed up at the beginning, consuming the wood greedily, then settled into a low, flickering, domesticated fire, then collapsed into itself, turning into glowing embers which brightened as the wind whispered or I stirred the coals with a stick.

Foremost of the silences I recall is our lying contented in one another's arms after sharing love—when words and lust are spent and the silence of certainty prevails. That, I think, must be the true secret of the biblical phrase "he went in unto her and knew her."

I will never experience such silences again because I have lost the one who knew how to spin the web of golden silence. Henceforth there will be silence, but it will be the silence of isolation and loneliness.

After pouring us both another cup of coffee, I glance at my watch—10:15. Kee needs to stay up a bit longer, so I open the *New York Times.* My desire to be well-informed, a desire which now seems useless and arrogant, has faded during Kee's illness, but I still subscribe. I want to be a good citizen, but making the world a better place is not something I'm likely to do much of now. Better to follow the Hippocratic oath and do no harm.

I scan the first section of the *Times,* collecting more details than I want to know about various horrors. Then I push the business section aside and pick up the section on science. Two articles on medical research interest me. Of course both are related to Kee's illnesses. Over the past eight years, I've read report after report of new discoveries and, less frequently, new treatments for Alzheimer's. What always distresses me is the frequency with which friends and relatives, catching a glimpse of a report in the newspaper or hearing something on television, jump to false conclusions about progress made. The public's gullibility is tragic. False hopes pile up on top of false hopes. The eagerness to believe in an immediate cure is fed by the media, not the more cautious scientists.

For a while there was talk about the possibility that aluminum poisoning caused Alzheimer-type dementia. Perhaps cooking in aluminum pans was a source of contamination. Later evidence indicated that the excess of aluminum in patients with the dementia might be the product rather than the cause of the dementia. But for a while, it made big "news." I suppose I should be sympathetic with the media as well as with scientists. They always confront the risk of being scooped by another reporter or news source. If it seems plausible, print it!

When I first read *The 36-Hour Day,* I was impressed with the care its authors took in describing the range of research on dementia. They held out no false promises and noted that scientists will pursue many research projects which will lead to dead ends. A long time ago I walked an enormous maze with our children. The density and height of the shrubbery made it impossible for us to know whether one passageway would dead-end or lead to another opening which, in its turn, would offer options, any one of which might abruptly terminate around a corner. We were fascinated by our failures and lost in the maze for almost an hour before finally working our way out. Only by going separate ways, then meeting back where we began and sharing what we found did we make our way outside the maze. That gives me a modest awareness of the mystery confronting neurologists, cell biologists, and epidemiologists as they pursue the cause of the widely varying symptoms evident in patients with dementia. As PET scans and MRI's provide more information about the brain and new drugs become available for experimentation, the possibilities and the potential dead ends before the researchers multiply.

This article on Alzheimer's disease at least raises no false hopes. It reports on progress in studying neurotransmitters. Already I'm out of my depth. I have at best a general sense of what a neurotransmitter is but have no understanding of their physical structure. And is physical structure the same as chemical structure? The article refers to acetylcholine. I haven't the foggiest notion what that is or does. Could I find out? Probably. Would that tiny shred of knowledge help me? Probably not. As a nonscientist, I live by faith. A passage in *The 36-Hour Day* describes how proteins provide highways through which chemicals travel within cells. I simply cannot visualize a chain of highways in my brain.

The only good thing I have witnessed in Alzheimer's disease is that it doesn't cause its victims physical pain. There are enough other maladies which provide pain. Astonishingly, the migraine headaches which troubled Kee for decades began to disappear with the onset of dementia. She rarely catches a cold. Although she has lost weight and was injured by her falls, she remains in what can be called "good health." That's ironic.

When I read reports about treatments which might in time be found to slow down the steady progression of Alzheimer's disease, I can only sputter, "Why, Why?" Why slow down such a terrible condition after the dementia once reaches the stage of diagnosis? Unless a cure is at least possible, slowing down the inexorable progress of the dementia seems hideous, as cruel and useless as using leeches to bleed a patient.

The article on cancer describes new methods of shrinking tumors by preventing the growth of blood vessels. Words like *endostatin* and *angiostatin* elude me, but the evidence on experiments with mice, according to the article, indicates that tumors deprived of access to blood vessels not only die as fast as they can reproduce, but, because they cannot reach other portions of the body, cannot metastasize. The article suggests that there is cause for hope of ultimately defeating the "Big C."

Somewhat cynically I read the article more carefully. Near the end of the item I find that the theory behind the research was first advanced more than a quarter century ago. What is new is the recent isolation of several drugs and some shifts in the attitudes of scientists toward the plausibility of the theory. The article does not mention whether any tests have been done with humans.

How many people will read this article or its reprints in other papers? Thousands, I suspect, will be calling their oncologists requesting treatment. I'm annoyed by the *Times'* misleading use of headlines which raise false hopes. Those I know who have died of incurable cancers experienced suffering worse than anything I've known. They endured full programs of treatments such as chemotherapy, radiation, marrow transplants, and other surgery. Some sought bogus cures in Mexico. Cheers for all the research, but I wish society would pay a little more attention to easing the suffering of those beyond cure.

Putting the paper aside, I look closely at Kee again. I say, "Hi!" and her eyes brighten and a trace of a smile shows. She raises her hand from her lap and I take it, holding it gently. Her other hand flutters impatiently. It dawns on me that what she wants is a cigarette. Releasing her hand, lighting another cigarette, I muse over the extent to which we live in separate worlds. I wanted a sign of her responsiveness and because I wanted that sign I misread her action. She simply wanted a cigarette. I did not understand. This is the reality of Alzheimer's dementia.

Kee is moving restlessly in her chair. Is she having a bowel movement? Her bathroom needs are unpredictable. Once she went ten days without a movement, and that was frightening, occasion for another call to the doctor. Not only was it distressing, it was a revelation. It's the only time I really wanted her to have a movement. The typical pattern for a BM is every other day, unless something causes diarrhea. The aides and I have a calendar on which all movements are posted. Although that sounds like an anal preoccupation, it's the only way I can keep the doctor accurately informed. From the calendar I know that she had a BM yesterday. It's neatly posted by one of the aides.

Early on, when she could still walk, Kee's problem was primarily with bladder control. As she became increasingly incontinent, I learned to be alert whenever she rose from a chair or from the bed. Sometimes she would get up and momentarily stand still as though thinking. Usually I would ask her whether she needed to go to the bathroom, knowing full well that there would likely be no correspondence between the answer and her need. A "Yes" or a "No" or a "I don't think so" was equally unreliable. But still I would ask, needing desperately to maintain some semblance of conversation. As I asked, I would also move closer to her trying to detect her next move. Sometimes after a brief hesitation, she would say, "I'm just walking," and then totter off, her weight too far forward as though she were preparing to dive into a pool. I would catch her by the arm and follow the direction she seemed inclined to follow, carefully maneuvering her around corners or chairs to which she seemed oblivious. As she became increasingly feeble, I taught her to place her left arm around my waist so that I could carry a portion of her weight on my hip. During our courtship and early years of marriage, our bodies seemed to fuse as we strolled forest path or neighborhood street arm in arm, each pliant and responsive to the other. In her illness, our movements became awkward, almost spastic. Sometimes we made a full turn through the apartment, but more frequently she would halt and look at me as though wondering why I was taking her on such an unnecessary and fatiguing journey.

Usually I would direct our course to the bathroom. If she protested and said, "I don't need to go," I would respond, "Well, it won't hurt to try," and she would meekly submit. At the beginning, I accepted too readily her assurance that she did not need to go. Moments later I might find that she had wet her clothes or even had a movement. The most unpleasant and distressing surprise I remember occurred before I started using slip-ons. I had called her to the telephone to say "Hi" to one of our sons. As she stood listening to him, she had a bowel movement in her underpants and was altogether oblivious to what was happening.

If I now ask her whether she is having or needs to have a bowel movement, she will likely say, "I don't think so." So instead I ask, "Are you ready to go lie down for a while?" "Yes, I think so" is the answer I expect and get.

I roll her wheelchair into the bedroom, lift her from the chair, and start to check the slip-on. It isn't necessary. An odor announces all that I need to know. Holding her close to me with my arms under hers, I maneuver her toward the bed. With one hand I grab a towel from a nearby chair and spread it on the bed where I will place her. Carefully, I let her sit down, then I lift her legs and rotate her into a prone position. With scissors I clip away the slip-on and reach for the role of paper towels. Toilet paper is inadequate for this task. Fortunately, the movement is not loose today. After wiping her buttocks with paper towels, I go to the bathroom, fill a basin with warm water, and get a washcloth. Had the movement been loose, I would need to give her a bath.

One of my major discoveries (Yes, even in so lowly a task a caregiver can take pride) was that when she had a bowel movement, I could place the disposable slip-on in an ordinary plastic bag from the grocery store. By tying the bag tightly and sealing off the odor, I could leave the bag in the trash can for hours before placing it outside to be picked up. Trying to wash the feces down the commode is both messy and laborious.

I confess that it has taken me a long time to become comfortable cleaning Kee after a bowel movement. Changing her when the slip-ons are soggy with urine never bothers me, but bowel movements are a different thing altogether. It's not the odor. I became accustomed to that when our children were in diapers. No, it's the invasion of privacy, the attempt to be impersonal, quasi-professional, in an area of physical intimacy. At first I also worried about infecting her and still have to be careful to be gentle when washing her. For a while I thought about shaving her pubic hair to make the task easier and cleaner, but I can't bring myself to do that. If you wonder why the pubic hair is a problem, just imagine having a bowel movement while sitting on a cushion.

It may be that one of my first experiences with Kee's loss of control affected my attitude, conditioning me quite negatively. Approximately a year following the diagnosis of Alzheimer-type dementia, I had to make an out-of-state trip. After checking airline schedules, I decided to drive. By then I couldn't leave Kee alone, and traveling by public carriers had proven difficult. On our trip back we had to make a daylong drive. For lunch I picked a motel restaurant. Before entering the dining room, I asked Kee to go to the bathroom while I did. She agreed, but when I came out of the men's room, she was exactly where I had left her. She said she did not need to go. Reluctantly, not trusting her judgment, I went into the restaurant with her, thinking that we could use the rest rooms after lunch. Until then, perhaps all would be well.

Before we were half through our meal, she said she needed to go. Yes, I was irritated, but I took her to the door of the rest room and waited. And waited and waited. After more than twenty minutes, certain that no one else was in there, I opened the door and asked if she were O.K. She answered, "Yes." From her tone I knew something was wrong. Hurrying back to the restaurant, I paid the bill, leaving the cold remains of our lunch on the table, then rushed back to the rest room. When she finally came out, I saw immediately that her pants were damp. I rushed her to the car, but as I helped her in, I noticed something on her right shoe. Checking, I found that excrement had flowed down her leg inside her pants and over her socks and shoes. She had lost control of her bowels before even getting to the rest room and spent so long there because she had been washing out her panties. Oblivious to the mess in her pants, she had taken them off to wash her panties and then put them back on fouled as they were.

There was nothing to do but take out a suitcase, take her back into the motel, and ask the woman at the desk to request others not to use the rest room until we came out. After washing her off and dressing her in clean clothes, clean socks, and a different pair of shoes, I thanked the desk clerk, tipped her too generously, and led Kee back to the car. Backing out of the parking space, I almost plowed into a parked truck. A minute later, entering the highway, I missed side-swiping a car hurtling along in the outside lane only by inches. The driver angrily shook his fist. That gesture and the scary near-miss made me aware that I was a cauldron of suppressed rage. I first became irritated when she did not go to the bathroom when I asked. I became more annoyed at having lunch interrupted. When I found her clothes covered with her own shit, I remained superficially calm, I think, as I helped her back into the motel and cleaned her, but I'm sure my teeth were clenched in rage. For four more hours of driving, I thought about the intensity of my anger.

Gradually I realized I was only mildly angry with Kee. Yes, she should have gone to the rest room when I first asked, but I already knew how little control she could exercise over anything. My fury was really ignited by the public humiliation I felt I had suffered and by my acute embarrassment. The fires of that fury were stoked by the eruption of the sense of unfairness festering in me. People routinely say, "Life is unfair." Then it seemed to me that the phrase conceals the truth that it may be outrageously *cruel*. And I was furious at life's cruelty. This was not what we had in mind when we planned for the "golden years" of retirement.

My rage, I think, arose from a deeper grievance. My companion, my friend, the woman I loved and shared life with had been robbed of intelligence and self-awareness. Even her loveliness was being eroded. My fury called out for an object of hatred.

As I attempted to examine my feelings, aware of the difficulty of complete honesty, I decided that the rage would never find its object—not God, not life, not someone or something. The hatred had to be dissolved and obliterated for me to survive, and I could think of but two solvents—thanksgiving and laughter. And both were as outrageous as the disease from which Kee suffers. I refuse to be thankful for something so destructive as Alzheimer's, yet there is a sense in which gratitude is involved. Not now. I'll try to explain that later.

Five years have passed since that dreadful day. Certainly I haven't eradicated the rage, but for the most part I have kept it tamped beneath the surface. Usually I manage to care for Kee with at least a semblance of poise and gentleness. But it's an effort. One day, not long after the falls which confined her to the wheelchair, she had three bowel movements in rapid succession, each following my re-making of the bed. I tried to remain calm with Kee—it was not her fault—but as I was placing the third load of sheets and clothing in the washing machine, the rage welled up. I wanted to punch some-thing or at least to scream out my grievances. Then I began to laugh, to laugh at my outrage, to laugh at my sense of being defiled by my wife's feces. I remembered a picture of a child playing in his own defe-cation, gleefully smearing it on a wall. Perhaps a small child could teach me, an old man fully attuned to the mores of a culture that treats bodily functions as unmentionable. What did I do to vent my feelings? What could I do? I added more soap to the wash and scrubbed my hands vigorously.

Now that Kee is thoroughly clean and has a fresh slip-on in place, I remove the towel and help her get comfortable. As usual, she says nothing through what in some way must be a terrible ordeal for her, too. Her eyes show discomfort, but she never says anything about her own humiliation or the indignity of being cleaned by her husband. If she did not have dementia, I would call her attitude one of denial.

I turn on the radio by the bed, tune it to the classical station, and say, "Rest well." She says, "I'll try." After kissing her on the forehead, my last action before leaving the bedroom is to gather up another dirty sheet and towel, then spray the room with Lysol, an act that always seems to suggest disapproval, but to that, too, she never re-sponds.

After shifting the first load to the dryer and putting another in to wash, I go back to the dining room table even though there's nothing there I want. This is one habit on which I can rely: go to the dining table, even if Kee is not there. But I don't want to play more solitaire and there's nothing I'm eager to read.

Over the last few years, I've begun to recognize that, at best, I have limited control of my thought processes. It's as though a part of me automatically dictates what I will do. I like to believe that to some degree I am independent of my mind, that I am more than synapses and currents. Maybe that's because I know that Kee *is* Kee although her mind has deserted her—at least mind in the sense that we normally use it. Of course I know that I cannot control dreams (which are always unruly succubi thrashing about to be born). Dreams happen. But in my conscious hours, too, I've found that I can rarely direct my mind along a straight path. My thoughts are like erratic "e-mail." What I "will" does not necessarily appear on the screen. My mind has its own ways, blustering into hidden, dusty closets that I thought long ago abandoned. Cobwebs and scattered fragments of the past whirl through my consciousness.

For most of my adult life I've been engaged in a flurry of activity, surrounded by people with whom, for the most part, I've pleasantly interacted. Some were friends, some merely acquaintances whom I encountered rarely, but I enjoyed the give and take—even with those for whom I felt no great warmth. From the flurry of activity I think I drew strength. A certain buoyancy arose from the sharing of responsibility and concerns. Coaches know what they are talking about when they demand teamwork. Now, here I am, stranded, confronting a weekend alone and very ambivalent about being alone. Why ambivalent? Because I don't want to be alone; yet, apart from Kee, there's no one I want to be with.

As Kee's condition reached the stage where others began to ask about her, I found myself uncomfortable even attempting an answer—except to our closest friends. Whatever I said was incomplete. Whatever I said might disturb or even frighten the kindly person who inquired. But I suspect it was embarrassment, too, that made me reluctant to talk about her illness. I was embarrassed by my own tendency to choke up. I was ashamed not of Kee's condition, but of my own inability to achieve some inner equilibrium. The deft control I had usually imposed over public displays of feelings deserted me. Gradually I shared less and less. Acquaintances became hesitant to ask anything, and I was grateful. Although I was warmed by the sorrow felt by our mutual friends, what I took to be obligatory expressions of pity from others irritated me. Yet I was also irritated if the conventional words were not expressed.

Even with our children I can rarely be completely honest. I tend to put the best face on things, to appear brave and confident even when I'm frightened and uncertain. I wonder if all the millions like me, dealing with the same problems day by day, feel as I do—alone, utterly alone, encased in a freezer to which I am self-confined.

When I first began to suspect that Kee's problems were related to Alzheimer's, I talked with a friend whose wife had been diagnosed with the disease a year or two earlier. He recommended that I read *The 36-Hour Day*. I did so reluctantly, hoping that it was not relevant to me. It told me a great deal about the clinical progression of the disease and about the demands confronting the caregiver. It was useful and sensitively written, but I also found myself resenting page after page. The authors brought ill tidings. My response was natural, if not kindly: "Kill the messenger."

They set forth the inexorable course of the disease, stage after stage of deterioration, clinically documented. Because I had no justification for disbelieving the authors, I was filled with unreasonable anger at their brief descriptions of what lay ahead. Merely by revealing my fate, the authors seemed accomplices in a cosmic, evil mystery. Even now, appreciative of the information they gave, I am not sure that I can forgive them. I have no Elijah to assure me that my barrel of resources will never be empty.

I learned to get through hours, even days, without succumbing to excessive stress, or so I thought. But as the full sense of what lay ahead of me unfolded, I began to see time as an enemy—not a personified enemy like the old man with the sickle, but a dark, marshy terrain stretching out beyond the horizon. I would be slogging forever through a waist-high swamp of minutes, hours, days, years. Mud would suck at my legs as I tried to move. In terror I would stumble, flailing at the malevolent algae clinging to me. I would grasp at branches which eluded me and strain to reach any position from which I could plot a course. Always I would fail. Yet failure terrified me less than the dark, slimy water. I prayed I would not drown.

In my thoughts I was eleven again and the submerged boat on which I played with my buddies had sunk beneath me. Sucked under into weeds and dark water, I panicked. For a moment, before thrashing arms propelled me to the dock, I feared I was drowning. The terror still lies deep in my bowels. Now, well over sixty years later, I live with the fear that I will be drawn into the darkness and slime again. I—we—must not drown. Do you have such fears? Yes, I think we all do.

Still sitting at the table, by habit I reach for the deck of cards. As my mind whirls through fears, past and present, a memory flashes into consciousness. Cards were involved in the first incident I can remember that led me to fear that Kee suffered from a dementia. When we were first married, I taught Kee to play bridge, which I had learned in the army as a cheap alternative to poker. Kee and I both took pleasure in the game, especially in the interdependence that partners share. We never became addicts, the kind who pursue every new system or cull the thousands of books and articles that might help them become better. It was merely a pleasant and cheap pastime.

When we were in graduate school, our friends were also poor. In the early years of our careers, we played with friends like ourselves who had young children and were hard-pressed to find babysitters even if they could afford them. Bridge was a satisfying solution. Children could be bedded down at the friends' home, or the friends could bring their children over. The games were friendly with long pauses in play for conversation. Rarely did Kee and I play more than six or eight times a year, but that was sufficient to maintain modest skills.

The memory is not dated, but the incident is vivid. Was it eight or nine years ago? Perhaps even ten? I don't know. What I do recall is the morning after a friendly evening of bridge, an evening cut short after four or five hands when Kee said that she did not feel well. The game had promptly dissolved. During the few hands that were played, I noticed that Kee seemed preoccupied. She reneged once and bid badly when she bid at all. That our friends had quickly won a rubber and were already vulnerable in a second when we quit did not upset me. I had learned long ago not to criticize Kee's bidding.

The following morning (we were on vacation), I asked Kee if she would like to review bidding procedures. She said yes, and so I dealt a few practice hands. Even after review, she seemed confused. I asked to see her hand. She showed it to me. It was not organized by suits. Some excellent players don't organize their hands, of course, but Kee was not among them. I suggested that she might find it easier to bid if her cards were systematically arranged. She looked befuddled. She no longer knew how to group the suits or arrange the numbers.

It was easier to give up bridge than to confront the significance of the incident. Perhaps she was just depressed. Perhaps her migraines were responsible; perhaps that evening she had had too much to drink. Perhaps—perhaps—perhaps. I didn't forget the incident, but neither was I able, at the time, to consider it in context with other failings. Later I told our children of the incident. They, too, ducked away from confronting the horror they feared.

Now the twelve cards, which bear age-old symbols of royal authority and power, seem to be judging me. Although they are only images on cardboard, they exercise power, if one submits to the rules of whatever game one is playing. A curious thought strikes me. In most games, as in bridge, kings, queens, and jacks are subject to aces. In poker two regal kings and two prancing princes fall before two aces and two pauper deuces. Man imposes the rules, but when cards are shuffled and dealt, chance determines fate.

Recalling the article I read earlier, I wonder whether scientists studying chromosomes will discover how genes determine a tendency to dementia. Once I read that genes from the father and genes from the mother can be distinctively imprinted. But *why* does one person carry a certain tendency and another person, no better, no worse perhaps, no poorer or richer, escape? Genes? Cold laws of probability? Fate? A malign force?

Maybe the depression so common to the caregiver arises from that conundrum. Why? Why me? Why mine? Why? I try to avoid such questions. I do not, will not, believe that Kee has been cursed by a sorcerer, much less by God or a demon. Yet she was smitten, struck down in what is so euphemistically called "an untimely fashion." Is no author of so great a tragedy to be located and blamed? In high school I stumbled across a poem entitled "Hap." I can't remember any particular line, but I remember my boyish shock at Thomas Hardy's fury toward the unknown and unidentifiable causation which he felt ruled his life. Unaccustomed to such belligerent accusations raised against God, I trembled before the blasphemy. Now I know what Hardy knew. Where there is no understanding, anger serves a useful, if dangerous, function.

Knowing that I will not get Kee up for a while, I decide I have time to check my e-mail. That I now use e-mail almost daily astonishes me. For almost a decade I resisted using this tool because of my distrust of machines and all things electronic. Now virtually all of my personal correspondence is sent electronically. I still talk on the phone with our children and a few local friends, but otherwise I punch in my message and, poof, it disappears into the ether.

Regular mail delivery is now something of a bore. I know its contents in advance: a bill or two, requests from three or four worthwhile charities beseeching generous contributions, an advertising flyer or two, and perhaps one of the three or four periodicals to which I subscribe. In moving from mailbox to the dining table (yes, I even go there with the mail) I detour past a trash can, pausing to throw out with relish advertising flyers and offers of more credit cards and to discard most of the requests for money, unopened, with some regret. As the expenses of Kee's illness increase, we . . . well, I . . . continue to contribute to the few causes we've supported for years, but I can't afford to add new ones. I've also discovered that a gift to a new organization promptly leads to more appeals from even more charities. It would be nice if they cooperated on each other's objectives as effectively as they share mailing lists, wouldn't it?

Turning the computer on, I nestle into my chair, waiting impatiently while electricity courses through the circuits. How it does what it does, I have no idea, but then I'm no better informed about my brain. As long as both work with modest efficiency, I'm content. I watch while the screen lights up and then goes blank. Messages, mostly warnings, flare across the screen, cute little hourglasses turn upside down, windows open on windows, various icons appear. Utterly amazing. When the screen calms down, I enter my e-mail system, obedient to its rules, click on files, and open my "in-box."

Two new messages have arrived since last night. One is a short message from our son in New York calling attention to an upcoming television program he thinks I should watch, the other a reminder of a meeting I unfortunately promised to attend. Just like the mail, not much of importance, but at least there are no bills. I've promised myself I will never pay bills by computer. I still want something tangible where money is involved.

Leaning back in my chair I ponder the personal computer, this miracle of my lifetime—not even my full lifetime, only its last few decades. In seconds I can send a message to a friend in San Francisco and, if the friend is plugged in, get a reply immediately. My grandfather would have hoped for a reply to a letter in several weeks, and his grandfather would have waited months, perhaps years.

In the file drawers of my desk are dozens of thick folders containing a portion of my correspondence and other papers before the advent of the computer and e-mail. Now a few discs can hold more files than this entire room can hold in their old paper form. In moments, through the little black box before me I can access all the messages I've sent and received for the last several months. To me that is a miracle. A new age, an age with technology I'll gladly use but can never master.

Since I have e-mail open, I decide to use it. I check the address file and decide to "hit" one or two friends to whom I've owed messages for a while. E-mail has not made me more punctual! Bringing up the address of a friend from whom I heard last week, I prepare to comment with appreciation on his note about Kee. I had recently declined an invitation to visit him and in the process spelled out more about Kee's condition than he had known. He promptly responded, expressing sorrow and concern. Now I find answering him very difficult. After writing a few sentences, I find that I've expressed one platitude after another. "I'm O.K. . . . The worst thing is that she is here but not here. . . . Coping with the loneliness is tough. . . . I can only take one step at a time." I stop typing. Pablum! Platitudes! Can I really say so little to people I care about? I try to backspace to clear the whole mess and begin over. The backspace glides over a few letters and freezes. I hit delete, then left arrow, then right arrow. The cursor remains stuck on one letter. Irritating. So, I joggle the space key a few times, then tab, then escape—nothing works. Irritation rises faster than a creek after a spring freshet. I'm exasperated. My impulse is to pound on the keyboard or smash the screen. Economic self-preservation vetoes those options. If something is wrong with my server rather than with my computer, I'll be shredding an expensive investment. I can either wait to see what happens or cut out. The decision is made for me. "Connection lost" flashes across the panel. I swear and turn off the computer.

Patience has never been one of my principal virtues. When I was young, whether playing basketball or organizing an event, I wanted action and results immediately. That impatience served me well as a student and, when I kept it in check, also served well in working with people. I once found a message I liked in a Chinese fortune cookie: "Consider the duck. Calm and collected above the surface, it paddles like hell beneath."

Where my impatience was most self-defeating was in raising our children. I had difficulty controlling myself whenever I felt they were "not trying hard enough." Quite likely that was the reason neither of my boys enjoyed sports and why my daughter's success came in ballet, about which I knew nothing. It took me a long time to recognize that all three were more patient with me than I with them—regrettable, unfortunate, but long, long ago.

When Kee's illness developed, "patience" took on new dimensions. Once the diagnosis of an Alzheimer-type dementia was made, some of my anger and irritability simply defused. Accepting the fact that no one is to blame, not even myself, I respond more sympathetically to Kee and look at my own behavior more objectively. That awareness and the liberation it brought, alas, has not suddenly transformed me into a model of patience, but it's a beginning.

Patience is undoubtedly a virtue for mankind in general, but for a caregiver, it is an absolute necessity. Without some measure of it, I could not survive. Yet neither can I deny my anger or suffering. The pain will not go away nor will the anxiety I always feel. Once I heard a sermon on "Blessings In Disguise." The thesis was that mankind is tested by God with trials and tribulations for the benefit of the sufferer—or sufferers. By such trials and tribulations one is humbled, becomes stronger, more Christlike. One should be grateful to be singled out by God for suffering. It made me remember the "Song of Bernadette" in which Bernadette (played by Jennifer Jones) is recognized as a saint not because of the voices she hears, but because the nuns discover putrefying sores on her legs which cause her excruciating pain that she bears quietly. A blessing from God? Nonsense. I didn't believe it then; I don't believe it now. Patience, yes, gratitude, NO.

I've tried to work out the distinction I'm making to my own satisfaction. To claim to be thankful for Kee's dementia would be hypocritical and self-deceptive. Giving thanks for all the good things experienced, for the love we've shared, for having spent more than fifty years discovering one another, yes, but there is nothing to be thankful for in dementia or cancer or AIDS or any of the myriad diseases besetting mankind.

Patience is an essential part of caregiving, yet a puzzling fact is that patience is easier in some relationships than others. When our children were small their needs were relatively easy to meet. Changing diapers, feeding them, helping them learn to read or ride a bicycle were things I could accomplish patiently. After they turned eight or so, it was a different matter. Yet dealing with my father in his old age was not too difficult. There, I think, I managed well—patiently.

The last trip I made with my father was when he was ninety-two, living in a retirement home. He was slipping into senility (or was it Alzheimer's?). Because he wanted to see some of his nieces and nephews and the old homeplace once again, I arranged to fly down to the retirement home, rent a car and make the long drive of some 225 miles. We had barely begun the trip when Dad said: "When we get there I want to see Ruth." Unfamiliar with the name, I asked, "Who's Ruth?" Dad explained that Ruth was Hank's daughter. I had at least heard of Hank, one of Dad's long-dead brothers. For the next five hours as I drove, every twenty minutes or so Dad expressed the desire to see Ruth. Each time I responded, "Yes, Dad, when we get there I'll find out where Ruth lives and, if at all possible, we'll see her." After the eighth repetition of this litany, I omitted "if at all possible."

When we finally arrived, I asked the cousin with whom we were staying if Ruth lived nearby and was told that Ruth would come over to see Dad that afternoon. When Ruth arrived, I met a vivacious woman perhaps twenty years younger than Dad. I could not recall having ever met her. Ruth led Dad into a corner where they chatted away for nearly an hour until she had to leave. When she left, I moved over to Dad and asked him whether he enjoyed the conversation. My father replied: "Who was that?" Unable to suppress the urge to smile, I said, "That was Ruth." Dad responded, "Who's Ruth?"

Why could I be cooly patient with my father yet have to steel myself to be consistently patient with Kee? Is the answer related to my father's age—or is it because I was rarely with Dad for more than a few hours at a time? I don't know.

It's possible that I'm a victim of my own expectations. If I press hard against rather spongy memories, I recognize that for years I anticipated Dad's aging and death. Although it was difficult to adapt to a new parent-child relationship after my mother's death, I gradually took responsibility for most decisions and all financial management until he died. I wasn't surprised when Mother died after a long illness at eighty-six or that Dad became senile in his nineties and died at ninety-five. It was fitting and natural that they should. What I did not expect was Kee's becoming totally dependent while still in the "good years" of her life. We expected to grow old together, sharing travel, books, music, friends—and now all of that is denied us. We knew that eventually illness would limit our activities but never anticipated losing the pleasure of sharing ideas and honing our perceptions and beliefs against one another's wit and intelligence. We never considered the possibility that one of us would live on and on in an essentially noncommunicative state.

Although four of our acquaintances developed Alzheimer's in their mid-fifties, we knew that most victims do not begin to show symptoms until their late seventies or eighties. Kee's gradual slipping into dementia was unnatural, unexpected, intolerable. Yet to tolerate it, or at least bring my own behavior into a more patient, gracious form is the task I face every day.

Dad has been dead for almost twenty years. I still am painfully aware that I did not do as much for Mother or Dad in their last years as I should, but on the whole I've accepted the restraints then limiting me, and I believe they understood and accepted the situation.

Memories of my parents, and of my older brother, who died before both of my parents, reinforce the sense of loss I feel in Kee's withdrawal into whatever world she now inhabits. To address issues tangled so deeply in my emotional life is not equivalent to solving them. Yet, sitting with this lifeless computer before me, mulling over the issue of patience, I realize how my attempts to be more patient are shaped by my anger, an anger which is real, deeply imbedded, even justifiable. But it is also destructive.

I do not fear becoming so angry as to harm Kee. I never have. My fear is that the anger, gnawing away in my gut, if unrestrained, unchecked, will eventually destroy me. To remain close to our children, I have to subdue the anger. I must rein it in to avoid losing friends, to avoid losing my own sanity. Above all, I have to flush it out of my system in order to like myself. If I can't like myself, I will never be wholly effective in caring for Kee. I probably will never altogether purge the anger, but by confronting it honestly, I might prevent it from destroying me.

To admit every day that I am angry and to remind myself that the anger still seeks an object is a form of therapy. I have to forgive myself for being angry. Sometimes I succeed. Just as often I don't, but there is consolation and hope in the effort. I try to be consistently patient with Kee. I try to be more accepting of myself.

Venting some of the rage is necessary. For me, the best purgative is violent physical activity, like playing handball or riding a bicycle as fast as I can. Yes, you are right of course. Drivers waiting at traffic lights do occasionally seem shocked to see an old man peddling madly past them. I like to think the gawkers are envious.

It's still a bit too early to get Kee up for lunch, but she might be getting anxious. So I limp down the hall to our bedroom. She sleeps lightly or not at all in the morning but likes to lie down. She is awake and seems comfortable. "You O.K.?" "I think so." "I'll come in soon and get you up for lunch, O.K.?" "O.K." "Call me if you need me." "O.K." It's what passes for conversation between us. I try to avoid intentionally inviting the response I want, but I fear I often determine her response by my phrasing or tone of voice. I've never heard of an Alzheimer's patient so affable.

Now I have time to write some checks. The checkbook in a desk drawer in my study is covered by a pile of bills carelessly tossed in when they arrived. Most of them are unopened. Why confront the reality before you must? Anyway, I know the approximate amount of each one. There is the monthly condo fee and eleven bills, including two from credit card companies, one from the electric company, one from the pharmacy, and one from the insurance company for a policy that supplements our Medicare. Others are from a department store, a dentist, a doctor, and Amoco. All of them routine, all the kind I've been paying from the beginning of our marriage, and all in the range expected. Early in our marriage Kee indicated that she didn't want to write the checks or keep our financial records. My guess, although I didn't tell her at the time, is that she didn't want me looking over her shoulder. She was right; I would have. I was far more compulsive about tracking finances than she was. One of our early spats arose from notations I made. As a kind of shorthand, I noted expenses such as "K's shoes" or, if they were mine, just "shoes." My explanation that I knew if they were my shoes didn't satisfy her at all. I changed my procedure and added "Burt's" when the purchase was mine. At the time that seemed preposterous to me, but I changed to avoid further bickering. Only in recent years have I begun to recognize that much of my behavior was, in critical ways, chauvinistic.

In a matter of minutes I've written, signed, and placed in their proper envelopes all but two of the checks. These bills, both from a medical supply house, are different—one is for the monthly supply of slip-ons, the other for the rental of her wheelchair. Although Medicare pays the bulk of the wheelchair costs, there remains some twenty-five dollars monthly that I must cover. The slip-ons bill, which includes the cost of the extra pads now used every night, runs in excess of a hundred and twenty-five dollars a month. If these costs and the cost of drugs keep rising, I'm fearful that we'll have to begin dipping into our savings—something I've steadfastly tried to avoid. At least we have some savings in the event our Social Security checks and my retirement check become insufficient. These thoughts, and they recur, lead me to wonder how caregivers less well off manage to make ends meet. Surely the anxieties and discouragement I often feel would be infinitely worse if our costs exceeded our income. I can see that day approaching.

The objective of keeping the savings untouched is to provide for the time, should it ever come, when I no longer have the physical and emotional strength or the mental alertness to keep Kee at home. I've visited several nursing facilities and am generally impressed with the quality of care given, but the costs of a very good nursing home are staggeringly expensive. I don't mean that they are excessively expensive for the service they deliver, only that most of us do not have the resources to spend fifty to sixty thousand dollars a year on nursing care. Anyway, I'm determined not to place her in such a facility if I can avoid it. The responsibility of caring for Kee is mine, and I don't want to relinquish it. Only if my health gives way will I resort to a facility for Alzheimer's patients.

My reasons for keeping her at home are no longer entirely clear to me. Initially her condition was not serious enough to justify placing her in a home. As her condition declined, I recalled a promise I had made to her years before that I would not place her in a nursing care facility unless I went too. There is the problem of cost, certainly, but the dominant justification is that I want to honor my promise.

I know that my desire to keep her at home has complex origins. Mixed into the issue somehow is my sense of self. I'm afraid that pride dictates much that I do. I need to prove to myself that I am strong enough to care for her. I want to be completely true to our marriage vows. Maybe these feelings spring from conceit or selfishness; I can't be sure. I do know that whenever I am forced to think about placing Kee in a nursing facility, practicality, idealism, generosity, and self-ishness become hopelessly entangled. I think it's more than being "old-fashioned" or superstitious about vows. I readily confess to bending truths or offering various misrepresentations. At the same time, I strongly believe that bedrock integrity is the greatest gift I can give myself.

How I argue with myself is a funny thing. Often I don't know which division of myself argues. Certainly I can't explain my inner arguments on the basis of that unidentified portion of self that makes judgments. Sometimes what seems to be selfishness argues for generosity; generosity might argue for practicality, which is the antithesis of generosity. Nevertheless, I try to isolate and identify the multiple divisions of self that I think I can recognize, or think I feel, or want to embrace as self. It's strange; I feel I am a relatively coherent self, but intellectually I can't work it out.

There was a time when these shifting, dyspeptic thoughts didn't plague me. I remember a dressing table in my mother's bedroom when I was a child. It had a fixed, central glass, larger than myself, with two side mirrors hinged to adjust to the light or the will of the viewer—a triptych of selfdom. Exhuming the scene from the rubble of memory, some lurking, pseudo-Freudian voice reminds me that it must have been my father's bedroom as well, but I can't imagine him looking into the mirror. Whatever doubts he had about his identity he walled off, I think, when he was ordained as a minister, and I never saw cracks in the wall. At least he seemed one and indivisible.

Another voice, less strident, less condescending, reminds me that the dressing table was also called a vanity table. I never think of my mother as vain about her appearance—vain in other ways, yes, as am I. As a child I loved to play with the multiple reflections, to lean into the mirror's embrace, to leap beyond it, duck in, duck out. Mirror, mirror on the wall, how many images can I call? Tongue straight out, tongue askew. Thumbs in ears, monkey face. Thumb on nose, you're the one. Smirking, giggling, hooking forefingers into the corners of my mouth, playing delightedly, not even thinking that I was playing with myself. The images were like playmates, magically conjured. There was no question then of images and reality. Like most children, I was so busy just being that I had no consciousness of being.

When did I first look into a mirror—eyeball to reflected eyeball—and ask "Who?" When did I lose the childish certitude that my image and my being were the same? When did consciousness raise the possibility of apparitions, of things superficially identical but unlike? I have no idea. Before photocopying, videotaping, televising, before we inhabitants of the twentieth and twenty-first centuries were inundated by a multiplicity of images, when did a child discover that the self he sees in a mirror is not the self he feels? When does awareness of duplicity enter consciousness?

As a preadolescent, I sought mirrors to discover myself, to imagine myself, to will self into being. As a child, my broad face with high cheekbones and light blue eyes conveyed innocence to others, and I was content with an image that rarely betrayed what I knew or, more particularly, what I had done. Teachers approved of me. I was chosen to play Papa Bear in the first grade; in the fourth, William Tell. Facing the classmate who played Tell's son, I propelled a suction-cupped arrow into the center of his forehead. Another classmate, playing the Austrian tyrant, laughed aloud. I've never quite forgiven him, but I have forgotten his name. The muffled snickers of other classmates and their parents stung my vanity, but I had been the star, however briefly.

When I was in the sixth grade, in a triumph of autocracy over democratic principles, the principal informed me that I was president of the school's chapter of the Red Cross. Furthermore, I was to give a speech to the P.T.A. I never knew, nor did I ask, why I was chosen or who prepared the lines I was to recite. Before a mirror I practiced childish gestures to emphasize the brutal treatment of animals in Hollywood Westerns. I gave the speech with sufficient fervor that the manager of the local theater was forced to pledge that he would pre-screen all Saturday morning Westerns to make certain that horses were not being pushed off cliffs or otherwise mistreated. Only twelve, I realize, and I was already accomplished in public fraud.

One is given a face—bones, skin, hair, eyes, the product of unemotional genes inexorably scripting outcome—and then one learns to shape the rudiments into a countenance that implies personality. He (or she) comes to know the face, to become accustomed to it, to use it, shaping personality and image simultaneously, to pretend that face, personality, and behavior are integrated. The face becomes a mask behind which contradictory impulses jostle one another for position and power. One is both casting director and actor.

Another memory strikes me, a memory of teenage years when I stared angrily at the image humiliating me, an image forcing me into a role I did not want to play. Grotesque pimples, pus-filled blackheads, globules of pestilence multiplied. Even my eyes and mouth seemed insufficiently attuned to my suffering. Acne was too kind a word for the ravaged, infested visage I saw in the mirror and detested. Even now, detecting evidence of scar tissue from the devastation of adolescence, I feel the self-loathing I experienced at fourteen, a self-loathing rising as spontaneously as the mysterious organ which welcomed me to puberty. There was no hiding, I felt. The appearance of celestial innocence succumbed to demonic forces. Beyond any control I could fathom, my body was quivering, pulsing, erupting, corrupting my very being.

Later there was the young soldier, untested by battle; then the avid student, perhaps less eager to learn than to impress his teachers; then the romantic courter of Kee; then the young husband and father desperately trying to live up to his understanding of what all of that meant; finally the profession I was engaged with for more than forty years as teacher and administrator. So who or what am I?

Technically I am a veteran altogether inexperienced in what a soldier is supposed to be adept in. I have degrees from distinguished institutions of education, but I am not sure that I am truly a dedicated student. I am son and father and husband, but I have never quite fulfilled my expectations in any of those roles. I have been honored as a teacher and an administrator, but often I have been more keenly aware of failures than of successes. I am a fraud who takes advantages of opportunities. I love Kee, my children, and many of those whom I've tried to serve, but do I have any greater love than that for myself? And I suppose what bothers me most is a tendency to behave arrogantly, to see myself as the center of the universe. Yes, who am I is a tough question.

Most of the roles I played, I chose, but the natural course of things sometimes overwhelms willful choice. So it has been these last ten years. I did not choose to become a caregiver. Yet I am determined to perform the role as well as I can.

Perhaps I spend too much time and energy in self-analysis. The more rational portion of my being warns me that I will never resolve such internal debates, but I cannot suppress the habit of self-examination—an examination biased by whatever mood I am in.

As I finger these last two bills, I think about how my own morale has fluctuated with every illness. The worst time was when I had the shingles. Then I was reduced to something close to hysteria, fearful that I would never again feel strong enough, physically or psychologically, to care for Kee. More recently the problems with my back and legs have reduced my general optimism. As when I had shingles, I have had difficulty sleeping. Some nights I try to lie quietly in bed while Kee sleeps, hoping that the silence will induce sleep. At other times, in the middle of the night I awaken with the leg throbbing and head to the kitchen for a snack so that I can take more ibuprofen.

There are times when I question my sanity. Can I really continue to care for Kee by myself for more than one hundred and thirty hours a week? And for how many weeks—months—years? Can I continue to afford the cost of the aides who provide respite for me for the other thirty hours? How long? How long can I last?

Still fingering the bills, turning them over in my hand as though I can alter them, I realize how much I miss talking with Kee about financial problems and plans. Although I kept the books and wrote the checks, she played an important role in any major financial decision. When major issues arose—when can we replace the roof, how do we meet our children's college expenses, when can we plan a trip, should we make plans for building a cabin in Colorado—I drew up a list of options and we sat down at a table to discuss them. Usually we came to an amicable agreement. Often she introduced options I had not considered which we adopted. Perhaps because her family was very poor when she was young, she was uncomfortable with large figures and preferred leaving investment matters to me. But I know widows who were left by their husbands without the slightest understanding of their financial situations, and at the time I was determined not to be one of the husbands who did so.

Then came the Alzheimer's. For a while I continued to review our finances with Kee monthly until one day she said, "I don't understand. Are we poor?" I reassured her that we were in no danger of the "poor house" as she remembered it from her childhood but that I did want her to understand the decisions confronting us. She said: "You make them."

Kee no longer has any idea whether we have a net worth of a thousand dollars or a hundred million. She seems no longer to understand the principle of costs. Since she no longer asks for anything, I confront the decisions alone. When we had to buy a new automobile, she seemed to recognize no distinction between that purchase and one of a loaf of bread. When we revised our living trusts, naming our daughter as executor and giving her power-of-attorney if I become incapacitated, Kee signed the document without question. In financial matters, too, I am alone, desperately alone.

Then I recall something of greater importance. Kee can no longer write her name. That crucial part of identity, asserting selfhood by writing one's name, has deserted her.

From the bedroom comes a cough—the sign that she wants to get up. Quickly I sign the two checks, place them in their envelopes, and try to seal off the thoughts that have distracted me. Such reflections, too, have become habitual. Nothing is ever resolved. My mind boils, and everything bubbles up briefly, then simmers down, out of sight, unresolved.

While asking Kee if she is ready for lunch, I move the wheelchair closer to the bed and let the side bars down. She raises herself on one elbow and says, "I think so." I help her into a sitting position and cut off the old slip-on. It's not very wet, but if I don't change her now, it will be much too wet by the time I take her back to bed. Anticipation is a great labor-saver. I slip on a fresh one and move her into her wheelchair.

In the dining room, after lighting her a cigarette, I ask whether she would prefer iced tea or coffee. This day she says, "I think coffee." I always ask, but it doesn't matter what I bring her. She doesn't remember what she asked for. One day, interrupted by the telephone, I poured her coffee before remembering that she had asked for tea. She accepted the coffee without hesitation. For several days I brought her what she did not request just to find out whether her choice had significance. It didn't. I found out what I wanted to know, but what good did that do me—or Kee?

I don't need to ask her what she would like to eat. In the early stages of the dementia, I tried to give her a variety of choices for lunch: cottage cheese, soup, fresh fruit, cheese, tuna fish. For the last several years, by refusing to eat anything else, she's made it clear that she wants only an open-faced chicken salad sandwich for lunch. I tested the chicken salad of four different stores and now drive extra miles to obtain the best. Making it myself, of course, is possible, but my chopping skills are so poor that it's not worth the effort. She will eat grapes or melon with the sandwich, fortunately.

I can't remember how long it took me to learn Kee's new signals in dementia, but it was a frustrating time. On some matters she would speak, even speak directly to the point. "No more fish" was clear; it did not require my interpreting body language. However, she rarely expressed such a preference or uttered verbal resistance. If she didn't want to eat, she clenched her teeth. Giving her a choice simply confused her. "Would you rather have chicken or roast beef?" was usually met with "That sounds good." Another standard response was "I think so," which helps not at all if the question is about what she might like for dinner.

Fixing her usual and a corned beef sandwich for myself takes only a matter of minutes. I add grapes to her plate, core an apple for myself, and sit down beside her. Trying to pace the feeding bite by bite to whatever rhythm seems to work best is often difficult. When she wants a drink of coffee instead of a bite of sandwich there's usually some slight gesture, but not always. Sometimes, she just closes her mouth.

Over the ten years we've lived in this apartment, the dining room has been the center of our existence. Kee may spend a little more time in the bedroom, but that time is entirely devoted to resting or sleeping. As her illness progressed, passion quietly vanished and with it physical intercourse. I continue to hug her, kiss her, fondle her, and her response is warm, but quite like that of an aging family cat who consents to petting. Why did we stop "making love?" (By the way, I don't really like that phrase. I think you share love; you can't make love.) Anyway, to answer the question, within three years of Kee's AD diagnosis, she was as limp when we had intercourse as when sitting in a chair. She showed no pleasure, and that led me to feel that I was abusing her. I couldn't live with that guilt, so we stopped "having sex." Do I miss sharing love with her physically? That's as silly a question as whether I am depressed. Aging does not completely eradicate desire.

It's the dining table that draws us together now. We sit together at one corner even when friends or the children visit. Sitting on her right side enables me to feed her more easily. Often we spend six or eight hours a day there. I may read her portions of the paper or passages that I like from magazine articles. In the mornings, she sometimes responds, by mid-afternoon, never. Yet I continue to talk with her of things I've done that day or of the whirr of imagination generated by words flat on a page. For my own well-being, I think I must not allow her silence to prevail, for I fear that silence will further unravel the bond between us. I dismissed one aide because she rarely attempted to initiate conversation, treating Kee as a thing to be watched rather than one to be loved as well as cared for.

Apart from that single incident, my experience with the women hired to look after Kee has been astonishingly positive. When Kee first showed signs of confusion and depression, I relied on a woman who had worked with us for fifteen years. She had come in only once a week to do some housecleaning, laundry, and ironing but was a close friend, particularly to Kee. They talked often on the telephone and visited one another occasionally. An older woman from Arkansas, she retained old customs, rejecting invitations to eat with us, but responding joyfully to Kee's banter (before Kee became ill) and their hugs before and after. As I grew reluctant to leave Kee alone, I arranged for the woman to come in more frequently. For several years I managed my schedule so that, with the housekeeper's assistance, Kee was rarely alone for more than two hours. With the diagnosis and steady progression of Alzheimer's, and the retirement of the housekeeper because of illness and old age, I needed more support, more for my own sake than for Kee's.

My first effort to hire a useful aide was unsuccessful, but then from a friend I obtained the name of a woman who did light housecleaning and who had experience with AD patients. I was less interested in how well she did housework than how she interacted with Kee. The woman was direct, cheerful, and energetic. From experience, she knew that she had to take the initiative with Kee. From the beginning she displayed an interest in Kee as a person, not merely a patient. That was what I wanted. I could do the laundry and cleaning, but when I was away from the apartment, I wanted someone who cared *about* as well as for my wife. One of the things that made me respond to her so favorably was the genuine interest she showed in Kee's former work. The woman agreed to come twice a week for four hours each day. I worked out the conditions of my last two years before full retirement so that I could be at home much of the time the aide was not there.

During the grim February when I was smitten with shingles and suffered from the ensuing combination of pain, sleeplessness, and deepening depression, I finally acknowledged that I had to have more help. I was learning slowly how far short I fell of being superhuman. One day I realized Kee had not recently taken a bath. I wasn't even certain how long it had been since she had bathed. I suggested that she do so and was ignored. The next day I said, "Love, you must take a bath." She responded, "I don't want to." "Would you like me to help you?" I asked. "I don't want one" was the stubborn reply. I insisted, leading her into the bathroom, drawing the water, helping her undress. Although I had read in *The 36-Hour Day* that bathing would become a problem, I denied that Kee was at that point. She refused to step into the tub. Irritably I picked her up, put her into the tub, washed and rinsed her now unresisting limbs and torso, helped her step out, dried her, dressed her in clean clothes, put her back in bed and went into my study and cried. If I was to survive psychologically, I had to forge a more normal life.

My options were limited. I reconsidered a nursing home but again rejected that choice. Not only was having a live-in aide beyond our means, but her presence would be an invasion of my privacy. I wanted someone to whom I could surrender responsibilities for more hours, but not permanently. From the Alzheimer's Association, I obtained the names of organizations which provide a range of choices for home-care assistance, from full time to a few visits a week. I selected one I knew to be reputable and agreed to a home interview by an agency supervisor. The interview's purpose was to assess the kind of assistance needed, to get pertinent background information, and to take a reading on the patient and myself. After working out an appropriate schedule based on my needs—two days for seven hours each—the agency informed me that if, for any reason, I was displeased with the first person sent, I should notify the agency promptly. Other candidates, previously interviewed, trained, and approved by the agency would be sent until I found one satisfactory for Kee.

From the moment I met the first young woman sent, I was pleased. She was an energetic young African American woman, quietly assertive and alert. She first sat and talked with Kee, not as though Kee were demented, but as if what was said was fully understood. Her touch was light and firm. Kindness and caring were evident. Without hesitation I left them together for three hours, returning at lunchtime. By then the helper had given Kee a bath, surveyed clothing and toiletry items, and become familiar with the kitchen. I left again, returning after another three hours to find the aide doing Kee's nails, something I had never done or even thought about. Kee was clearly responsive to the woman, smiling and enjoying her new companion. I felt a momentary pang of jealousy because Kee was responding to this stranger as warmly as to me.

As the young woman left at the end of her first Tuesday, she inquired whether she should return on Friday, the date scheduled for the second visit. At first I misunderstood her, thinking there was a problem with the day of the week. Not so. The young woman was politely asking if I wished to retain her. Since shortly after her arrival, it hadn't occurred to me that I could find anyone better. She has become indispensable.

Now for more than three years I have relied heavily on these two generous women with confidence that they care deeply about Kee. In personality they are quite different. One is almost boisterous and enjoys teasing, the other more serious, more empathic. I trust them both and am grateful that they have become part of my family. I can leave home certain that all Kee's physical needs will be met, and, more important, that she is with someone who senses that, had Alzheimer's not struck, they might have been friends.

I don't think it was sheer luck that I hired them, although I was lucky that they came along when they did. When she was healthy, Kee had an intuitive sense of people, of what their motivations were, of what they sought. I think she taught me some of those skills. In our first interviews I sensed that these women possessed the virtues I primarily wanted: patience, empathy, and reliability. They've more than confirmed that impression.

While these thoughts run through my mind, I continue to feed Kee, watching for signs that she is ready for another bite—occasionally taking a bite of my own sandwich. I may break the silence to ask, "Is that good?" or "Would you like some more coffee?" or to warn her that I am about to use her napkin to wipe her chin. I've learned to be careful with motions that might startle her. When she finishes the sandwich, I ask, "Would you like a piece of cake?" To that she responds, as she often does: "That sounds good!"

Kee's delight in cake matches her pleasure in a morning pastry. Do you think the addiction to sweets is a kind of throwback to childhood? My father's favorite food in his dementia was ice cream, and the problem was withholding it from him until he finished his meal. Kee rarely eats ice cream and doesn't particularly like cookies. Ah, but pastries and cake! The problem with cake is finding a variety that doesn't adversely affect her digestion. Chocolate or caramel cakes almost always produce diarrhea. Usually I hunt for split lemon or a lightly glazed bundt cake. In a pathetic effort to control my waistline, I try to avoid cake, but then gorge myself on cookies.

Clearing the table after lunch, I realize there is something missing in my self-flattering review of success with home-care aides. I haven't given credit to the person most responsible, Kee. Early in her illness, a doctor told me, "The mind goes but the personality remains." I question whether that is always true. In fact from other caregivers I've heard of disruptive changes in behavior. In the later stages, some Alzheimer's patients with no previous history of violence become belligerent, attacking nurses and loved ones. With rare exception, Kee remains sweet and gracious.

One thing that intrigues me is that, during a mid-stage of her disintegration, she often responded to a friend's innocuous "How are you today?" with "Mean as ever." I've joshed her about that, suggesting that she needs to practice her "meanness." She never makes the connection between her assertion and my teasing. She is merely baffled. But what prompts her perception that she is mean? Is it only another automatic phrase? Is it possible that part of her wants to scream and strike out at anyone or anything, that at some level of being she is sternly controlling those impulses? On the other hand, I have a vague recollection of her telling me long ago that her paternal grandmother, who *was* mean, greeted her visitors when she was past ninety with "I'm mean as ever." So perhaps I'm reading into Kee's behavior my own response to the devastation of AD while she is simply mimicking her grandmother. I'll never know but am profoundly grateful that if she has any impulse to attack me, she effectively squelches it. I don't know how I could possibly survive hostility.

So often I want to know what goes on in Kee's mind. Does she know that she is usually sweet and gracious? When she acts confused, does she know that she is confused? Is her "Mean as ever" an effort at humor? Sometimes I feel that she is coyly playing cat and mouse with me. I hope not, but can I truly know?

I think it's important for a caregiver to think about such things, to prepare for the unknown, anticipating what may happen. But then a caregiver, like an Alzheimer's patient, is distinctive. Each of us must work his or her own way through the swamp.

My watch says 1:05. I am, unfortunately, compulsive about time. If I'm not wearing a watch and don't have access to a clock, I feel uncomfortable. Kee has long since escaped that prison. Whether it is 10 A.M. or 10 P.M. makes no difference to her. Although her body retains some biological rhythms, her mind is simply not attuned to time. Around twilight, she becomes more confused than normal. I had read of the "sundown effect" and seen it represented amusingly by an actor on a television show, but it is not amusing to discover the vulnerability of one's wife to the pattern.

Her need for sleep does follow a definite pattern. Generally she sleeps well from about 11:00 P.M. until about 8:00 in the morning. I'm fortunate in that. When she returns to bed later in the morning and afternoon she doesn't sleep. Those are "rest breaks." She might close her eyes, but I never find her asleep then.

Why I continue to be so compulsive about time I can only guess. Keeping a schedule has been habitual most of my life, of course, but there may be something else coercing me to keep things scheduled. It's like trying to impose order on chaos, to give life some modest definition. I may also be trying to measure out how much time remains, how much longer my sentence before I leave this prison behind. At my worst moments, I feel that the sentence was unjustly pronounced. The trial was held in my absence, and I was given no opportunity to plead my case. There is no one to whom I can appeal. Has the prison been more unfair to Kee or to me? It doesn't matter because fairness plays no role in such matters. Further, I know that the imprisonment was not imposed on me as it was on her. I chose to care for her through this ordeal. Nothing outside my self would have prevented my walking away, going to the Bahamas to laze in the sun or to Alaska to chill out. I chose to serve my time, and it remains the only option for me.

My watch still says 1:05. Almost ten hours remain this day. About 3:00 I will take her back to bed for an hour or so. About 5 P.M. I will start supper. Soon after that we will have a drink together. Then we can string out eating and sitting at the table for another hour and a half or so. About 8:00, I'll take her back to bed for another hour, then wheel her into the family room and turn on the television. She won't watch it, but we'll be together. Lately, however, she has quietly protested against going to the family room, preferring the dining table. Does that preference relate to how much attention I give her in one place rather than the other? I don't know. It may just be that she finds the incomprehensible action on the TV screen and the sudden noises issuing from it unpleasant.

While she rests in the morning, in the afternoon, and after dinner, I usually retreat to my study. There I keep up communication with friends or read. I treasure those minutes, and I also usually stay up for an hour or so after she goes to bed. That's "wind-down" time.

The hours most difficult for me to get through are the hours immediately after lunch. She wants me by her and doesn't want me deeply involved with anything else. Two or three years ago, sitting with her after lunch, I often read, but fiction drew me in so that, engrossed in my reading, I neglected her. The newspapers or magazines I read after breakfast do not demand a lengthy attention span. They also rustle rather pleasantly and lead me to make observations. When reading a novel, however, I am far away, and she resents my absence as though I were the one who had deserted her.

One day after lunch, shortly after her diagnosis, I was rereading Dickens' *The Old Curiosity Shop* and cackled out loud. She was so startled that I tried to explain why I laughed. Trying to explain humor is always a grievous mistake. I had decided to read the book because it contains an old man becoming progressively more senile, a personal fear that has developed in my less settled moments. I soon became bored with Nell and her grandfather. Nell was too goody-goody (the perfect little caregiver), and the old grandfather was little more than a stock figure arousing no interest.

But Quilp! The rediscovery of Quilp perfectly suited my irascibility. No other character in fiction so thoroughly embodies unrestrained malice. I had felt dark, clotted malice rising in my own spleen. Not directed at Kee, not directed at anyone or anything, just the desire to lash out, to be destructive, if only in imagination. And Quilp's malice is presented in a hilariously comic manner. I need the laughter as much as some outlet for anger!

I came across a passage in which, with "uncontrollable delight," Quilp plies one of his victims with fiery whiskey, completely addling him. In spasms of delight, Quilp rolls on the ground. Then, just beyond the reach of a dog, he dances demonically, taunting the cur while it leaps ferociously against its chain.

Unsuccessfully I tried to explain to Kee why I found the scene so funny. I haven't convinced you either, I see. Anyway, I explained that in creating Quilp—that ogre, that dwarfish giant of a character— Dickens acted out his own frustrations and desire for vengeance. Dickens couldn't behave like Quilp, but while writing he could *be* Quilp. Drowning Quilp at the end and driving a stake through his heart would be penance enough.

As a reader, I experienced the vicarious delight that Dickens felt. I know that I would detest Quilp if he were real, that I would find him repugnant, but there is a delight in destructive behavior—in throwing off self-imposed inhibitions.

Hours spent playing with my grandson have reminded me of the joy of destruction. Together we painstakingly construct elaborate castles out of building blocks, but the boy's greatest pleasure comes in smashing our constructions with a toy truck. I remember similar delight when I was a child. The building of a sand castle was an excuse for jumping on it. Model airplanes were built so that they could be held out the window of a speeding car until the wings came off and the whirling little metal propellor wore right through its pin. I could also tell you of schemes of vengeance I have imagined, particularly toward my army drill sergeant. The joy of destruction, the delight in outrageous malice! I can relate to that, but I couldn't explain it to Kee. You still don't see the humor? Try reading it. Dickens does it better.

I'm glad that my anger over Kee's illness hasn't led to some act of public outrage. The deep-seated anger does make me crabby and crotchety, however. Sometimes it makes me wish that I were a little boy who could gleefully lay waste to something. An act of wanton destruction might bring relief. But there is nothing to do, no *thing* to hold liable, except life itself. If imagining destructive, malicious vengeance is a sin, I fear I am unrepentant.

Yes, the musings I allow myself are often weird. So is my sense of humor, twisted as a stick of licorice made of black bile.

I reach over and take Kee's hand, as though apologizing for miscreant thoughts. She looks up and smiles.

Coverage of a PGA tournament comes on the television at 2:00. I want to see part of it, and if Kee is not too tired, she will agree to be moved into the family room. She won't watch the screen but will sit quietly, smoking whenever I allow her a cigarette, drinking another cup of coffee and appearing to be deep in thought. Golf on television disturbs her less than football, basketball, or hockey, where the speed of play and the excitement of the crowd produce a state of semiconsternation. When I turn on golf, I try to keep up the illusion of conversation. If I say something like "Did you see that shot? or "Ooh, he missed that simple putt," her response, when there is one, is usually "Yes, I saw that" although her eyes have not once lifted toward the screen. Still, I like for her to be with me and can't leave her alone at the dining table.

She does not protest when I wheel her into the family room. There I arrange a small table near her chair for her ashtray and cup. Often she forgets to tap the ashes off so I have to be alert to keep her from dropping hot ash on her clothing.

Shortly after marrying, we agreed that golf would be a pastime we could enjoy together. Neither of us wanted to spend large portions of our limited free time pursuing different pleasures. Unlike some couples, we did not need a reprieve from each other's company. Golfing together was an attractive choice, although Kee was no athlete. She could neither throw nor run well. She grew up at a time and in a place where strenuous physical activity was considered "unladylike"—unless, of course, it involved chasing after children, doing the laundry, or, in hard times, picking cotton.

After a brief trial in college, she gave up tennis as too exhausting. Fishing did not appeal. Golfing, she thought, would suit her slight frame and purposeful temperament. I agreed enthusiastically, envisioning years of contented scrambling over golf courses together.

I hoped we might be able to find the time (and the money) to play once or twice a month. One of her friends, quite a good golfer, took her to a range and instructed her on a grip, the basics of the swing, and the rudiments of club selection. That was more instruction than I ever had. The first few times we played together, she struck the ball well—better, more rhythmically than I did. She couldn't hit her tee shots far, but her lazy iron shots from the fairway had a nice loft and fair distance, although direction posed problems. I also noticed a distinct problem when her wedge traveled as far as her five iron. She (and I) found this tendency annoying when she was thirty yards from the green. She crossed back and forth over several greens four or five times before picking her ball up. But she said nothing. Not one of the many appropriate expletives passed her lips. I sensed our golfing together would be short-lived.

Over the course of that first summer of golfing together, we went out several times. On our third effort, she quietly insisted on a golf cart. No more strolling together down the fairway. On the fifth green, a two-level monster with undulations like a troubled sea, she concluded that four putts was both a reasonable and maximum number for each hole. Henceforth, she would remove the ball from the green after that number, no matter where it lay. I offered no objection.

The first time we played on a weekend, I became uncomfortably aware that her twelve to fifteen strokes a hole, coupled with my own six or seven, required significantly more time than that consumed by the golfers in front of us. As that foursome vanished from sight, I saw that the foursome behind us seemed to suffer from St. Vitus' dance. I suggested to Kee that we needed to speed up play. With annoyance, she responded that she couldn't hit the ball any faster. I withheld my thought related to distance. We finished the round not as jovial companions but in a simmering stew.

The following year, whenever I suggested that we play, she urged me to have a good time, making it clear that she would forego the pleasure. She found the weather either too hot or too cold. I soon came to recognize that "just right" meant seventy-two to seventy-five degrees with humidity no higher than 50 percent, a climatic condition that occurred in our home area once in a decade. Then came the children, and neither of us had time or money for golf. Occasionally I would manage to play once or twice a year.

Many years later, while we were camping in Wisconsin and the children were taking a canoe trip, I persuaded her to go out with me once more. The day was gorgeous, meeting even her conditions. Through the first six holes, she tried gamely to appear interested. On the fifth hole, a par three, she ran a long chip in and for the first time in her life broke seven. On the next hole, however, after advancing down the fairway about 150 yards in only three strokes, she made a smooth swing on her fourth shot, but hit it off the toe into high rough. I made a brief effort to retrieve it, but by now the foursome behind was becoming restless. I waved them through and cautioned Kee to be alert while we watched from the rough. The first three hit excellent shots down the middle, more or less where my ball lay after two shots. The fourth to play hit a low screamer in our direction and bellowed "Fore." I saw that it was slicing toward us and warned Kee. She responded by turning her back. The ball struck thirty or so yards short of us, bounced several more times, and took a nasty carom directly toward her, nicking her in the calf. She was not seriously hurt, but the sudden pain increased the gross sense of indignity she felt. Someone was shooting at her.

When the gentleman who hit her arrived to play his second shot, she ignored the savage's profuse apologies—and never played another hole. Thereafter when I wanted to play golf on vacation, she would drop me off at a course and go antique shopping. The cost of the two ventures came close to balancing out. Over the last two decades, she has encouraged me to play at least once, sometimes twice a week during the summer months, but I always thought her encouragement lacking in enthusiasm—unless a new antique shop beckoned.

I had hoped in retirement to play frequently, perhaps even to take lessons, maybe take a few strokes off my handicap. When her dementia was diagnosed, I grudgingly gave up such hopes. Not until our children recognized my need to get out of the apartment and I hired the aides did I begin to play more frequently. Then came my back injury, weakened legs, and despair. Soon, I hope, I will be able to get back to the challenge golf offers . . . well, to some of us.

To play great golf you need to start as a youth and play frequently year after year. When I was a teenager, part-time jobs, including delivering newspapers at six A.M., deprived me of the luxury of time. Nor could I afford to purchase clubs or pay greens fees. Even later, after being mustered out of the army, I was able to play only three or four times a year.

I am not a "natural." My swing is unpredictable. I top drives, watching the ball bound erratically a hundred yards or so before dribbling into a depression. My iron play is more encouraging but never more than a fraction away from an errant slice. Short chips become short chunks. At any moment I expect an angry groundskeeper to rush up and beg me to play elsewhere.

In spite of my flaws, I pursue the game with the intensity of an addict seeking heroin. What I need to do, even at my age, is take lessons and develop the fundamentals of a good swing. Reason makes its plea: "Take lessons." The hacker in me says, "Play, you can do it." So I play, badly as well as infrequently, but with the forlorn hope of becoming sufficiently adept that I will not always embarrass myself. For nearly forty years I have tried to translate what I read about golf into what professionals call "the mechanics" of the swing; yet my swing never gets beyond the beginning erector-set level. My failures don't send me to a professional; they lead to more reading, processing information which I comprehend, but which my recalcitrant muscles steadfastly ignore. My head bobs up and down, my knees buckle or lock at precisely the wrong moment. I can't effect a good hip or shoulder turn. Lunging at the ball plagues me. And still I play whenever I can. In rare moments of sanity I acknowledge that for me a bogie is a victory, a par an unexpected joy, a birdie to be dreamed of, and an eagle part of mythology.

Do you play golf? No? Then I fear I am boring you. Be patient. Golf is an instructive game. Yes, golf draws sneers from some (although I never heard anyone sneer at a professional golfer who earns $350,000 over four days), but for others it has a magnetic attraction. Part of its draw, I suppose, lies in the fact that the game does not require a particular physical type. You may be short or tall, thin or heavy. I have been out-driven, out-putted, out-scored by all physical types, both men and women.

Watching professional golfers on television delights me because there I see what I know I am supposed to do yet can rarely accomplish—the smooth swing with perfect synchronizing of hands, arms, shoulders, hips, and legs at the precise moment of contact with the ball. At times, of course, to watch the "pros" is intimidating. One look at Tiger Woods and I knew I would never swing a club or anything else so powerfully. I get whiplash from watching him.

The best golfers, whatever their styles, have certain traits in common, including patience, persistence, imagination, and an extraordinary ability to concentrate. I will never combine such traits into a unified whole. What keeps me going is what sustains the average hacker—credulousness. For duffers and hackers like myself, credulity is the greatest quality of all—the faith that the next time out, the kingdom of par-shooting will be entered.

The qualities I've ascribed to great golfers apply equally to caregivers, and I fear that my caregiving skills, like my golf game, need much improvement. Consider the following essential traits:

Patience. Whenever I become angry or overly expectant, inevitably I fail to meet Kee's needs. On the golf course if I have an "unfair" lie—the ball rolling into a divot or into a tuft of grass on a badly mowed fairway—I can move the ball and pretend I'm playing "winter rules." In helping an Alzheimer's victim, you can't change the "lie." You accept things as they are or fail. If on the golf course you shank or top a ball, anger has to be swallowed down or it ruins your next shot. If I spill something on the sheets or break a glass trying to help Kee, irritation will ruin the rest of the day—for both of us. Patience, self-forgiveness, accepting what is and what lies ahead: there lies salvation. Anger betrays both patient and caregiver.

Persistence. I remember Lee Trevino saying that anyone could become a good golfer if he hit three hundred balls a day. I doubt that, but my failure to practice, to repeat the same stroke over and over until my muscles are programmed to the correct groove will always prevent my achieving a low handicap. Trevino-like persistence requires the willingness to sacrifice everything else to master the game of golf. Once I honestly accepted my role as caregiver, sacrificing virtually everything else became inevitable, but the price was high and consistency difficult to achieve.

When I chose to care for Kee at home, I could not imagine the demands. I survived the first few years by sheer persistence. Trevino could set three hundred practice balls a day as a standard. There are no numbers the caregiver can formulate. Slip-ons must be changed. Dirty clothes pile up if unattended to. Soiled beds to clean, laundry to do, medicines to give, meals to prepare, spills to be mopped up— these represent the lightest portion of the load. What requires the greatest effort is remaining calm while responding to Kee's unpredictable behavior. In trying to anticipate the unexpressed need, I burn energy as though it were limitless. In trying to avoid treating her as an infant, I consume irreplaceable emotional resources. When asked by a considerate friend how I am managing, I have no satisfactory reply. Any reply seems either trite or self-consciously heroic. Persistence, easy to define, is exhausting to realize. Yet in some strange way, persistence creates its own energy.

Imagination. On television I've watched great golfers come up with shots I didn't believe possible. After hitting an errant drive, one "pro" hit his second shot through a minuscule opening in the branches of a tree; another curled a shot entirely around a tree; yet another putted fifty feet through the rough cut of an oddly shaped green and sank it. Imagination has played a very modest role in my attending to Kee, but that's probably my fault. A practical nurse suggested that I place less food on Kee's plate to avoid overwhelming her. It worked, and occasionally she indicates she wants more. I had difficulty keeping the laces of her shoes tied. Since she can't manage them at all, I solved the problem by shifting to slippers.

When incontinence first became a problem, I found that diaper-like underclothing annoyed her and made her even less likely to use the toilet. By observing closely and making mental notes, I discovered that she might go several days without soiling herself, but once she did, there would likely be frequent instances immediately following. I learned to use slip-ons only after the first incident and to begin each day with normal cotton panties. That worked until the falls that confined her to bed necessitated the constant use of slip-ons.

Before becoming bedridden, she had difficulty dealing with dresses when using the toilet. I simply shifted to soft sweatpants, which were easy for her to manage and for me to wash. I discovered that what I supposed to be her craving for alcohol rested principally upon thirst and taste. I satisfied both and solved the problem of too much alcohol by giving her a glass of water with only a tablespoon or so of scotch in it, and repeating that two or three times each night.

One other trait of a good golfer is relevant to caregiving, and it involves a contradiction my body cannot cope with on the golf course—concentrating intently while remaining physically relaxed.

I know that too tight a grip on a club creates tension throughout the body, yet, when concentrating on my swing, I hold the club as if I have broken through ice and am desperately clinging to a tree limb held out by a would-be rescuer. I know there are those who have the knack of swinging fluidly while taking into account lie, distance, angle of execution, and bounce. I am not one of them. Water hazards reduce me to the state of a terrified child confronting a third inoculation. When considering a simple five-iron shot over water: wild-eyed I clutch the club in a viselike grip. Inevitably what follows is a constricted swing, shoulder dips, hip wiggles, head bobs, and combinations thereof which defy the imagination. After dousing the first ball, I am likely to introduce exaggerated variations of the same flaws on the second shot with the same result.

That same tension, the same sense that I can accomplish something better by trying harder equally plagues my efforts at home. I am close to being a "control freak." At work I was sometimes congratulated for being well organized in a tone that implied more. I did like things in order; I liked to count on results being predictable. I planned vacation trips with the exactness of mock military maneuvers, making reservations at motels days ahead of a trip, calculating miles traveled, rest stops, sightseeing excursions. At work I initially confronted tasks with pencil and paper. List upon list of things to accomplish and the sequence in which they should be done followed. The addiction to order and control inevitably produced tension. I sometimes required hours to unwind from travel or work. Occasionally I developed tics in my eyelids. In sleep, my legs twitched.

Maybe, maybe what I've learned from caregiving will someday carry over to my golfing. It's too late to be of use in my vocation. I now know that rigidity, particularly rigidity with schedules, dooms effective caregiving. If a bath is needed, it can be given sometime in the course of the day, not necessarily at 10:05 A.M. Nothing can be planned with precision. I depend on time measurements; Kee no longer understands the concept of time. Constant referral to my watch is as absurd as it is useless. When I used to help Kee to the toilet, if I was tense, that tension carried over to her. Relax! It really doesn't matter whether she takes her medicine at 9:00 or 9:45. I do not run a hospital. Acting like a martinet is foolish. Relax. I am trying to reduce my compulsiveness about time. Relax. An easier swing increases distance.

In a way I'm embarrassed by these somewhat farfetched analogies between an activity I thoroughly enjoy, golf, and an obligation to which I have committed myself. I do enjoy caring for Kee some of the time and being with her much of the time. However, I hope never to hear anyone claim to enjoy every moment of giving care to one they love. To make such a claim would require elements of sadism, masochism, and dishonesty. Which, do you think, would predominate?

That brings me back to the word *credulity*, which I used when I was listing the qualities of a golfer. I guess it doesn't apply to *good* golfers. And for hackers like myself, credulous isn't quite the right adjective.

Perhaps gullible comes closer. A good golfer *knows* he can hit a given shot. If he needs to carry 140 yards, bounce the ball off a mound, and let it feed into the pin, he believes he can do it. His confidence arises from having done it many times before. For the hacker, who has never succeeded in such a shot, to attempt it demonstrates gullibility. The slogan "Play within yourself" simply hasn't registered. He wants to succeed and thinks there is an outside possibility that he can. He swings, watches the flight of the ball, and grinds his teeth, cursing, as it dives into a sand trap.

The frothy gullibility of "maybe I can" never quite conceals the hard-rock probability of failure. Whether blasting out of a sand trap or hitting off the tee, the hacker distrusting himself fails. Disbelief guarantees failure. The slightest uncertainty produces muscular response—too much or too little wrist, too much or too little hip action, loss of balance.

As I've aged, the inability to maintain my balance has plagued my golfing. Similarly a failure to achieve balance—emotional balance—may be my greatest shortcoming in attending to Kee. Over the course of any day, I veer from pleasure at our still being physically together to despair over her loss of sentience and the absence of any foreseeable end to my duties. I try to convince myself that the duties are opportunities, chances to show love and appreciation.

When, for a brief period, I do achieve that belief, I clean, wash, cook, bathe her, and talk to her without condescension, even with enthusiasm. But maintaining such conviction as a constant state of mind has proven impossible. Frankly, I get tired.

My worst times are when I feel indifferent, as if an alien being consumes me, a creature who can sympathize with neither Kee nor me. At such times, I feel anesthetized, sloshing mindlessly through the swamp without purpose, unable to praise or pray, only to suffer with no assurance of survival.

There are times when I want to repeat all that I've done for her over the full course of her illness, certain, or at least hopeful, that I could better express my love through caregiving. If I could go back nine or ten years, would I make the same choices? Even if I could go back and relive these last ten years with Kee, golfing has taught me that the same foibles and follies would plague me. Just as there is never an absolutely perfect round of golf, I would never become the perfect caregiver, though I had twenty such challenges.

I wonder, in fact, if I am being gullible in thinking that I can sustain caregiving for so many hours for an indefinite number of years. Am I imposing unreasonable demands on myself? At times giving up seems attractive. Then credulousness, which has positive as well as negative qualities, sings out: "I'll do better tomorrow. I'll feel better tomorrow." I continue to return for round after round. Trying somehow sustains me.

Preparing to light another cigarette for Kee—the last one before taking her to bed for her afternoon rest—I recognize an unmistakable odor. That she can sit calmly in her wheelchair and have a bowel movement confounds me. Before her dementia led to complete incontinence, she had been almost prissy about bodily functions. From childhood she was modest and intensely private. Now she seems unaware that she is having a bowel movement or, if she is aware, unable to admit it to herself.

I wheel her into the bedroom and move her to the bed. From the case covering her wheelchair pillow, which is messy, I know that I'll need to take her into the bathroom and give her a complete bath. Giving her a tub bath is something I do reluctantly and infrequently. One of the women who helps us is much more efficient and at ease with her, so I take advantage of those skills, bathing Kee only as necessary on the weekends.

The bathing, too, has a history. I've mentioned that in the early stages of her dementia she resisted bathing, but after her falls, I found that the task became quite daunting. A month or so after her second serious fall she had a very messy bowel movement on a weekend, when I was alone. A washcloth was totally inadequate. Although the practical nurse was scheduled to come the following day and would bathe her, I couldn't wait. To get her clean required immersing her lower torso.

By that point in caring for her, I had learned to try to think everything through in advance. She had not been out of bed since the fall. She would not be able to sit up in the tub without support and would resist lying down. I would have to get in and cradle her between my legs, washing her by reaching around. Because the bath in the guest room was larger and could accommodate both bodies, I decided to use it. I knew that the tub's shower doors made maneuvering difficult, but I assumed I could manage. The bath was a necessity.

The first thing to do was draw the water—warm, but not hot. As I drew the water, I reminded myself to take a change of clothing and new underpants for her into the bathroom before picking her up (I had not then obtained a wheelchair). Girded with what at the time I thought a meticulously developed plan, I told her what I was going to do, going over the details. Her eyes registered suspicion, but no terror. Then it occurred to me that it would be easier to remove her gown before taking her to the tub. As I slipped off her gown, I realized that once I picked her up, I wouldn't be able to put her down until we were both in the tub. No choice; I undressed, giving thanks that our windows were ten stories above street level.

Carefully, I bent over the bed, drew her toward me, bent my knees as much as the bed allowed, and lifted her. This was no time for my back brace. I knew that carrying her to the guest bathroom would tax my strength, but what else could I do? For the first time I realized that I had to get a wheelchair.

I started toward the door. As we passed the bedpost, she seized it while I was in midstride. I almost fell but managed to pivot around without dropping her. "Let go! Let go of the bedpost," I said. Her grip tightened, her knuckles whitening. She hadn't held anything so tightly in three years, I thought. "Please, I'm afraid I'll drop you. Let loose!" Not a chance.

Using her firm grip as one stable point, I managed to get my right foot up onto the side rail of the bed, rest her against that knee and pry her loose, moving her still-grasping hand to my arm. Lifting her again, I tottered off toward the bathroom, praying that I could still manage the twenty-five or so steps ahead of me. A weird thought popped into my head—*Candid Camera*—lurid shots of two seventy-plus-year-old nudes staggering down the hall past woodblock prints of Japanese noblemen peeking at us from their frames on the wall.

In the bathroom I carefully put one foot into the tub, maneuvering Kee's body so that I could swing her in without smashing her against the door. Dammit, I had forgotten that I threw out the old rubber bath mat several weeks earlier, intending to replace it. With no traction, I was afraid of slipping and both of us taking a nasty fall. Keeping one leg outside the tub, I rotated Kee into position and placed her on her right leg. Because of her injury, the left leg couldn't take the pressure of her weight.

I asked her to hold onto the rail fixed on the inner wall. She didn't understand until I showed her, and even then her grip had lost the force so evident when she seized the bedpost. Only when I brought my other leg into the tub did I realize that my plan overlooked critical details. Could I loosen her grip and let her down slowly into the water? Should I sit down first and pull her down onto me? I tried the former, but she almost slipped below the water surface and began to panic. I drew her back up, let her take another grip on the rail and sploshed myself down. Now, how to get her to let go of the rail? Using my most gentle, reassuring voice, I begged her to let go and trust me. Even with dementia, she was too alert for that.

I rose on one knee, loosened her grip, and gradually let her down, this time managing to hold her head high enough that she did not panic. The problem was that I was in a kneeling position. There was no way I could straighten my leg out. Oh yes, maybe if I were twenty-eight, but I wasn't. Quickly, I soaped a washrag and began bathing her, letting her head and torso lean against my body.

My leg began to cramp—badly. But if I stood up, she would slip down. Moving as rapidly as I could, I cleaned her bottom, upper body and thighs. There was no way I could reach her feet. The cramp was becoming worse. I began to laugh, not quite hysterically but uncontrollably. "Roll the cameras," I snickered. "We're starring in our own farce! Are you having a good time? Do you wanna do this again tomorrow?" Her answer was terse—and, as stage directions would note, "with feeling": "NO." There was no "maybe, maybe," no "whatever," no "I think." It was a simple, effective declaration.

I tried to rise from my kneeling position to ease the cramping and lost my footing, coming down behind her with a splash but still holding her up. Her hair was drenched, and I had no intention of giving her a shampoo, not in that water. But at least my leg was straightened out and the cramp disappearing. Now what? I couldn't risk the chance of her slipping and falling. For me to rise from a sitting position while holding her up seemed impossible. Time for ingenuity. How would the Druids at Stonehenge have solved such a problem? Ah! Incrementally.

With the aid of her natural buoyancy, I managed to lift her from between my legs onto my lap. Then with both hands under her buttocks I raised her just high enough so that I could get my knees up and let her sit there briefly while I shifted my hands from lift mode to push mode. The objective was to get her to the point where she could hold onto the rail. Placing my right hand under her right buttock while holding her steady with my left, I shoved her higher, imploring her to grab the rail with both hands. She missed. We tried again. This time she succeeded. Continuing to push with the right hand while guiding her with the left, I got her into a crouching position, hoping she could hang on. As quickly as I could, I pushed myself up, nearly falling again because I couldn't reach the bar and dared not grab her. I was still laughing and beginning to think I was hysterical. Steadying myself, I placed one foot outside the tub, grounding it on a mat, and lifted her. She would not let go of the bar. I jerked her loose.

Safely out of the tub, I placed a towel on the commode, sat her on it, and dried her with another towel. She was shivering. Her eyes were unforgiving. Was she distressed by my clumsiness and her understandable fear or did she find the laughter humiliating? "I'm sorry, love, but we had to do that" was all I could say between spasms of laughter. I then put clean underpants and a gown on her and carried her back to bed. She immediately soaked the underpants, the gown, and the sheets. I quit laughing.

Oddly enough, I find this memory amusing and satisfying. Recalling it several days later, I was able to objectify the situation, to see it as an observer rather than as a participant would. The capacity to stand aside after the fact has been a saving grace for me. It has turned intolerable situations into satisfying memories. It enables me to laugh at my own incompetence. It allows me to tell our children and close friends what is happening without crying.

Now bathing Kee is much easier. After the "*Candid Camera* scene," I reread the section in *The 36-Hour Day* on bathing. Now we have the wheelchair, the rubber mat in place, a shower hose, and, perhaps most important, a specially designed chair for bathtubs. I also removed the shower doors from Kee's bathtub so that transferring her from the wheelchair to the tub seat is much easier.

To wash her properly, I still find it easier to undress myself and get into the tub with her, but that is no longer really necessary. I can place her on the chair, test the water from the hose, spray her thoroughly, and, using a soapy washrag, clean her as well as if she were sitting in a foot of water. Keeping the bathroom warm enough to avoid chill is the only difficult task.

Even now, bathing her is not a speedy operation. By the time I have her bathed, clothed, and back into bed for her rest, it is almost four o'clock. And now there is another load for the washing machine.

I've completely forgotten about the mail. On Saturdays the time of its arrival is always uncertain, but rarely is it delivered later than 1:00 P.M. I'm not expecting anything in particular but feel obliged as a good American to do my duty. Do you think other cultures are as dependent on the idea of mail as is my generation of Americans? When I was a boy, if the mail was late, the ensuing family irritability could lead to a crisis. Rarely was anything of significance expected, but delayed mail seemed to suggest a tottering government. Did the Postal Service with its slogans about sleet and snow create this phenomenon?

The ritual nature of daily mail, Sundays and holidays excepted, seems deeply planted in the national psyche. Even as the writing of letters declines, replaced by telephone and e-mail, it seems to me that expectations of some unanticipated delight from the mail remain high. I had a colleague who expected the arrival of the office mail at a precise time. If the mail was delayed, he became angry, pacing the floor until the opportunity came to berate the mail boy. If there was nothing for him, he was only mildly annoyed. What was important was that the mail arrive on time. On federal holidays, when there is no mail, good citizens of sixty or more have a queasy feeling of emptiness. My children don't seem to suffer from this very odd affliction.

The ritual of punctual mail service was implanted in my mind with sound and visual effects. Each summer in my boyhood I went with my mother and brother to a rustic cabin, owned by an aunt and uncle, in the lower reaches of the Appalachians. The cabin had been built by my uncle and his son. Rustic was a code word for unfinished. Cheap lumber, thoroughly soaked in creosote, was overlapped and supported by two-by-fours. Unpainted two-by-sixes held up a tarred roof which had to be retarred every two or three years to reduce the number of leaks to a tolerable level. At night, after a heavy rain, I was lulled to sleep by the steady drip, drip of water into metal pans, a sound mingled with my uncle's snoring. The four rooms were unfinished and drafty. The rafters supporting the roof slanted up to twelve or fourteen feet while the partitions separating the rooms rose no more than eight feet. It was, one might say, a companionable setting. To the best of my knowledge, no children were ever conceived there. The openness of the upper area provided a kind of contraception by public exposure.

The largest of the rooms had an enormous stone fireplace. I remember watching the shadows of a fire flickering on the roof over my bunk at night. With judicious use of wall spaces and bunks with ladders, as many as fourteen persons could sleep there, if they had no compulsive need for privacy. Plumbing and electricity were not introduced until the very late 1930s. A path led to a one-seat outhouse about thirty yards away, a path one was loath to take at 3:00 A.M. My uncle, a resourceful man already in his late sixties, kept a chamber pot by his bed.

The pride of the cabin was the spacious front porch, which offered a sweeping view of the valley and the mountains beyond, a panorama any landscape painter would covet. In the late afternoons, clouds and sun washed the mountains with variant blues and purples. Some days you could see the rain coming from the western sky, moving like a curtain across the valley until the thundershower drenched the cabin.

The immediate setting was as rough as the cabin. No effort was made to clean out underbrush. Vines twisted and snarled through trees. A hundred yards below the cabin was a creek which trickled down the mountain on which the cabin perched. I liked to trace the course of the branch to its beginning in a small spring, climbing up through blackberry briars, ferns and rhododendrons, scrub oak, pine, and the occasional chestnut to an outcropping from which I could see the blue ridges stretching into the haze beyond. Because my brother was five years older and had his own interests, I usually climbed to my retreat alone. I sat there, tossing stones and fantasizing about myself as a twentieth-century embodiment of Daniel Boone or Davy Crockett.

The cabin was some mile and a half from the small village which provided our mail address. The valley, known for its beauty and a boarding school for mountain youth, a school that later gave the world *Foxfire*, extended some forty miles from north to south. An ancient railway line with equally ancient and dangerously decrepit wooden trestles connected the valley to the rest of the world. The train, which ran from south to north in the morning and returned in the afternoon, was sole custodian of the U.S. Mail. The old steam engine chugged its way through the valley, the engineer jovially tooting at every crossing of a country lane. Given its age and the condition of the track, the train, consisting of the engine, one passenger car, a mail car, and the traditional red caboose, was astonishingly punctual, arriving at the village daily about 11:45 A.M. and returning about 3:30.

My daily chores were not demanding. My principal responsibility was to set out for the village, rain or shine, as soon as I heard the whistle of the morning train. If it was raining, I preferred to go barefoot, feeling the mud oozing up between my toes. Through the woods I followed a path which led to an unpaved road lined with pastures, fields of cabbage and corn, and the occasional run-down shack. By the time I reached the village, the postmaster would have sorted the mail, lit his pipe, and opened the general delivery window.

The mail sometimes consisted only of a newspaper, two days late, sent up from the city. Occasionally there was a letter from my father or a note from another relative, but the point of my going for the mail was less related to its contents than to fulfilling the sacred obligation to get the mail. Returning to the cabin, I often walked along the tracks paralleling the country lane for a quarter mile. If I was barefoot, I walked the rails. Shoes were less suitable to the game, which included counting the number of cross ties passed before I began to wobble, lose my balance, and slip off the rail. The newspaper served as my balancing stick. If I was bringing home milk, always in glass bottles before the days of cardboard cartons and plastic jugs, I was under strict instructions *not* to walk the rails.

Some days I was entrusted with money for bread, milk, or eggs to be bought at one of the two tiny, but fiercely competitive, general stores, each featuring identical flour and pickle barrels, enormous boxes of crackers, and tantalizing jars of penny candy. My aunt, a "furriner" to the mountain folk, was fully aware of the impossibility of protecting the cabin during the winter months. As insurance, she wisely divided her business between the stores since the respective owners both had relatives and in-laws populating most of our area of the valley. Her policy worked better than State Farm. Over thirty years, the cabin was broken into only once, and then the only thing stolen was an utterly irresistible fishing rod which should not have been left there.

Those memories are unique to me, and I hope never to lose them. I once took Kee and our kids to the cabin, but they couldn't really share the experiences and certainly not the warmth that accompanies them. They were not deeply impressed by the remnants of the concrete fort I had once built for toy soldiers, or by a yet-standing, forked stick I set by the branch to hold one side of a flutter-mill. I, too, was disappointed. The one paved road of my boyhood, which ran the length of the valley, had been straightened, widened, and regraded to meet the needs of the diesel trucks, tourist buses, and sleek automobiles that now tear along the road at manic speeds. The train has long since vanished; only the tracks lie there as a memorial to a time past. More disheartening is the smoke spewing out of new industrial plants, plants which have displaced the pastures, the cattle, and the fields of cabbage or corn. Now Kee probably doesn't even recall going there, and as far as I can tell, she has little or no recollection of events in her own childhood. To lose one's memories is to lose the life one has led. I would prefer death to the loss of my memories.

Was life better when I was a boy? No. I recognize nostalgia for what it is and innocence for what it used to be. At nine I was not aware that we were living through a depression. Where I lived, most people had been poor since before the Civil War. The mountaineers were just more so. They farmed small plots of string beans, tomatoes, and sweet corn, kept chickens and hogs, hunted squirrels and possums, and sat on their porches plucking guitars or playing mouth-organs. The more entrepreneurial kept stills, hidden well away from their cabins. Later, during the forties, they found the black market in sugar and gasoline more lucrative.

If life was not better when I was a boy, neither was it worse—just different, incomparably different. For a child, it moved at a slower pace and depended less on manufactured stimuli. I didn't see my first movie until I was five. In 1939 we went to the World's Fair in New York and there saw an experimental television presentation, but we never dreamed that within a few short years this miracle would be available to a mass market. In my boyhood, evenings were for reading, for games, for chasing fireflies, or for watching stars from the front porch while the adults chattered. How will my children feel at seventy, looking back on childhoods marked by frequent travel over long distances, by vicarious television trips to the moon or the Serengeti, by the living room immediacy of Vietnam and the drug culture? I only hope that some of their memories of childhood will enrich their lives as memories of my childhood have nourished me.

Why have I tried your patience with these memories? Forgive me. I know you can't truly share them. But you have your own memories, recollections that partially define who you are, what you have been, even where you will go. Our ability to recall the past, both the good and the bad in our lives, accounts for our sympathy for victims of amnesia. Memory softens us, hardens us, opens us to new experiences, closes us to what we fear. I've read articles and sections of books which contend that Alzheimer's victims are blessed by their inability to remember. Such nonsense infuriates and nauseates me. Without memory, what are we?

As I reach for the few envelopes, fliers, and magazines in the mail basket, I notice two letters of solicitation addressed to Kee. Even letters from old friends are no longer addressed to her. Except for computer-generated mailings, only birthday or Mother's Day cards bear her name. Within a few years, even that will end; Kee might never again receive a letter. Never! And soon her name will disappear from magazine subscriptions and mailing lists. The finality of so trivial a matter is unnerving. I feel once more aggrieved—and lonely.

From the window of my study I can see the tops of apartment buildings to the west. Absentmindedly I gaze out the window, focusing on nothing, as I put bills in the drawer where I keep my checkbook. Perhaps an apparition might appear. The sun is moving toward the horizon. A few clouds seem to gather there. In a few seconds my eyes blink as a pigeon flutters into view. It settles clumsily on the nearest roof and walks across it splayfooted, not pigeon-toed, bobbing its head as though greeting unseen friends. Clearly an individualist.

How old is it, I wonder, and what is the normal life of a pigeon? Pigeonwise is he, too, a septuagenarian? Has he lost his mate? And why have I labeled a bird of undetermined gender a he? But I know the answer. I now tend to look at most things from an egocentric point of view. But I'm not really thinking, I'm just pasting verbal tags on what my eyes register. Verbalizing perceptions is itself a habit. I'm amused that I have used "pigeonwise," part of the growing tendency to make everything, and nothing, "-wise." Somewhere, someone is probably saying "moneywise." Has anyone yet used "truthwise?" Possibly. That certainly will precede "deathwise."

The pigeon, slate gray against the tarred roof, pauses, craning its head back in my direction. At this distance I can't tell if it winks. I have the suspicion that the bird looks toward me with Quilplike malice, as though it is plotting the terrible vengeance at which pigeons excel. Although of the family of *columba,* this is no dove of peace. Yet it seems free, unburdened by any obligations.

I want to get out, to go for a walk, to breathe fresh air, to feel the cooling breezes of late autumn. Two years earlier, without hesitation, I would have told Kee that I was going for a short walk and would, in good conscience, have left her alone for thirty minutes to an hour. I had different walks for every time span.

Leaving my study, I move into the living room so that I can look out over the park. My favorite walks, when it was possible to go out, carried me through different sections of the park. The park is an old friend. During the past forty years we have never lived more than a mile away. Now the trees in the park seem to beckon, waving their branches gently as though urging me to join them.

When we first came to this city and were close to the poverty line, we rented an apartment with no air-conditioning. Fortunately, the stifling heat of early September soon gave way to the pleasant temperatures of the fall. The following summer, however, the heat struck early and ferociously. We could not afford to buy even a window air conditioner for the bedroom. A floor fan purchased at Goodwill for five dollars offered little relief. In the early evening, when the outdoor temperature still hovered in the mid-nineties, and the buildup of temperature in the poorly insulated apartment became nearly unbearable, we sometimes put our two toddlers into our decrepit but dependable Plymouth and drove the half mile to the park. If there was no breeze, at least moisture from the trees cooled the air.

Sometimes we took a small portable grill and cooked hamburgers when three pounds of hamburger cost only a dollar. While I prepared the grill and Kee organized condiments and buns, our boys rushed about, making the discoveries that only children make—an oddly shaped twig, a snail, a wildflower, a stone. After eating burgers, Kee and I rested on a blanket or tarpaulin, enjoying the children and one another. Late in the evening, usually well past our boys' normal bedtime, we reluctantly returned to the apartment and a sweaty, half-sleepless night.

The park gave pleasure to many people and served as an equalizer. A picnic table was available to the first person who claimed it. Wealth and status made no difference. I have, I believe, shared the park with virtually all nationalities, all races, all religions. All claim the park as their own; all seem prepared to share it with everyone. It is the kind of place that gives one hope for and confidence in democratic ideals.

Gazing aimlessly but wistfully across the park, my hand touches a bird's nest sitting on the windowsill. It reminds me of a walk I took about two years ago. Perhaps I remember it so well because at the time I knew I would not have many more spontaneous walks, walks taken as the mood hit me. It was a special occasion.

After crossing the thoroughfare and climbing the slope leading to the first range of trees, I noticed this nest about seven feet up in a lower limb of a young tree. Obviously it wasn't a sparrow's nest; it was a work of art. I studied the twigs and strands of grass which were skillfully woven together to form a small basket lined with mud and then relined with a mixture of soft materials. It was cemented to the branch by a mud base. How many months had it been exposed to the winds and rain? One of nature's marvels. The birds who constructed this wee abode had no degrees in architecture, no blueprints to guide them other than what nature inscribed in their tiny brains. I had read that birds who make such nests peck up dirt, then regurgitate it to form the mud which seals their nest together and to the tree. Incredible.

I wasn't sure what kind of bird built so compact and refined a nest —a thrush, perhaps? I fingered it gently and decided that on my way back I would detach it and carry it home. I wanted my grandson to recognize the beauty of the work and the miracle of its making. Perhaps even Kee would enjoy it. My grandson's first impulse might be to smash it, but he might also recognize something of how nature works and be encouraged to treasure it. Briefly I thought of leaving it on the limb, but, imagining its destruction by winter storms, decided that an unnatural setting was better than that.

Marking where I would find the nest on my return, I strolled through undergrowth toward a distant path that led deeper into the woods— the John F. Kennedy Memorial Forest. Its few inhabitants are squirrels, rabbits, warblers, jays, robins, ravens, an occasional flicker, and the usual array of sparrows. These woods lack the range of bird life of the high Rockies, where on any walk I can see vireos, orioles, nuthatches, and Western jays and where nighthawks fill the evening sky. When I was a boy, I occasionally saw tanagers. Not now. Even butterflies seem less common and less varied in species.

As I walked toward the forest, I wondered why starlings, grackles, and pigeons preferred to build their nests in the crevices and eave supports of the apartment buildings a few hundred yards away. While habitats for warblers shrink, grackles fatten and multiply in "civilization." In spite of the sporadic efforts of a few environmentalists to protect remaining stands of forest, habitats keep shrinking. Perhaps only the naming of this portion of the park as a "memorial" will enable it to survive.

What will I do when Kee dies? How can I best celebrate her life? Maybe having trees planted within our view of the park would be good.

She wouldn't care about a piece of stone or a bronze plaque beneath the trees so that others might identify the donor. Living trees would suffice. Perhaps the pair of birds who built the nest, or their descendants, would be drawn there. Memorials do not have to be publicly proclaimed. Probably not one in fifty of those who walk these woods know they memorialize JFK. By the year 2050, only a few outside the context of a classroom will recognize the initials. I rather like the fact that flora and fauna are unaware of mankind's need to memorialize itself.

The path I followed winds through thick underbrush, fallen trees, vines, and briars. Over them a canopy of branches and leaves rustle and darken the path. This part of the park is left untended deliberately. Not having been prettified, these few acres do not attract many. Only twice have I encountered people on the path. An occasional plastic cup or crushed beer can nevertheless proclaims that these woods are not mine. Once I asked a young man not to throw an aluminum can into the woods. Looking at me quizzically, the young man handed me the can, saying, "You won't get rich off that, pal." At least he felt a wee sense of communal bond even if our assumptions differed.

The canopy of branches and leaves was opening up. The annual splendor of reds and oranges had given way to dry brown, and the path was strewn with signs of retreat before the harshness of winter. During winter months mud and slush transform the path into an obstacle course I have never challenged. But I don't see fallen leaves as signs of death. They are promises that the rich canopy will form again in the spring. Although I have had neither time nor energy to walk that path in the last two years, it comforts me to know that it has changed little and that I may yet walk it again.

The path ends at one of the macadam roads curling sinuously through the park. I chose to turn left, a route that took me up near the museum and toward the golf course. Paralleling the road is a path for roller-bladers, cyclists, joggers, and pedestrians. As I walked the path, cyclists calling out "left" whipped past before I knew they were coming. Hearing the approach of roller-bladers, I stepped aside, feeling a kind of kinship with them all. Lovers strolled through an open field. In the spacious open area in front of the museum, four children and three adults were flying kites. One of the adults, an expert, was alone. His kite soared far above the others, and the twine remaining on his spindle gave evidence that he was accustomed to its reaching great heights. He gave the string a slight tug, and his kite dipped in recognition.

The children varied in aptitude. One boy, perhaps ten, had gotten his kite up but was having difficulty managing it as it swerved and veered beyond his control. Another boy, no more than six, was making halfhearted attempts to get his kite to rise as a man, presumably his father, shouted encouragement. The lad was game but had not learned how to let out the string. As he ran into the wind, the kite trailed behind him, bouncing in protest.

A bench at the top of the hill was the ideal place for me to sit and watch. The child who could not get his kite aloft stopped to watch the expert. I wanted to explain to him that the expert had gone through all the stages of kite-flying himself, had rushed about with his kite ricocheting off the land, had dealt with kites which mocked him, had achieved his skills only through failure. The boy's father encouraged him to try again. Father and son reminded me of my failures with my children—always trying too hard to get them to succeed, not content to let them learn from failure.

Tired of being the bystander, I arose from the bench where I'd stopped to rest, glanced toward the kites and their would-be masters, and turned toward the golf course. I knew few would be playing at that time of the year and day. Older players prefer the early morning. Because daylight saving time had ended, men and women who worked normal hours would not be able to squeeze in a round after work. But there was nearly always someone playing—a few school boys who rushed to the course after the final bell or college students without late afternoon classes. Because this was a public course, all manner of attire and quality of equipment appeared. The variety of skill was even greater than that of dress.

This day a young African American, playing alone, and unaware of my presence beneath a nearby oak, had the thirteenth hole completely to himself. He took several relaxed and rhythmic practice swings, lined up, and ripped the ball toward the green—a beautiful shot. As it does on instructional videos, the ball rose on a line down the middle of the fairway, soaring toward the horizon as if free of gravity. When it finally struck the ground, it continued on a straight line, bounding, bounding toward the green. The drive covered more than 280 yards, a distance I sometimes do not reach in two. The young man held his swing, statuesque, as though modeling for a sculpture in a Greek stadium. When the ball stopped, he brought the club to his lips, kissed it, then lovingly placed it in his bag, tapping it fondly. I continued to watch while the golfer strode briskly toward his ball. He chose an iron, again took several practice swings, lined up his shot, and lofted the ball toward the green some 130 yards away. Even from my position, I could tell the shot was true but long. I waited until the young athlete completed the hole—a short chip, a putt, a par—and moved to the next tee. Rarely on my walks did I see such skill, such assurance. I felt that the young man, his tools, and the course respected one another, uniting to elevate a skill to an art.

The bird's nest, the kites, the skilled golfer—memories I continue to hold close. Yet as I look out now, what strikes me are my thoughts about the canopy of fall leaves soon to give way, first to barrenness then to recovery in spring foliage. And beyond that the canopy of the sky, it, too, subject to change from sullen clouds to pelting rain to puffs of cotton clouds against peaceful blue sky to blistering sun. The cycles of nature, relentlessly changing. And, like most of mankind, I find myself stubbornly resisting natural changes as I age, seeking to elude the inevitable.

I surrender the pleasures of reverie and return to my study. The sun, just over the treetops, blazes through the window, daring me to stare it down. I draw the blinds, but not before noting that the pigeon has gone its own way.

By now Kee is probably restless and ready to get up. When I look into the bedroom she rises on one elbow. I don't need to ask whether she wants to go to the dining table to have a cigarette, but I do anyway and receive the usual "I think so." I put her into a fresh slip-on, then, bending my knees, I help her to stand, and carefully shifting my feet, slide her into the wheelchair. Suddenly, like a child with a toy car, I make a roaring sound, call out, "Fasten your seatbelt," whip the wheelchair around, angle through the doorway, and swoosh into the dining room. I'm not sure that she likes this playful gambit, but she says nothing, and I feel better for making a momentary game of it.

After lighting a cigarette for her, I get her a glass of ice water with a straw before sitting down next to her. She manages all liquids better with a straw. I'll fix our drinks in a few minutes, but not until she has had several glasses of water. The water is good for her and, by quenching her thirst, slows down her consumption of the little alcohol I'll give her.

Just before dinner has always been the time when we unpacked the baggage of our days, sharing incidents and concerns over a drink. Before moving into the condo, if the weather was good, we sat on the patio of our home for this ceremony. Although Kee never shared information about her clients, there were always my encounters with colleagues to talk about. And I could speak openly about students or administrative matters which were not confidential. Or we might talk about the need to do something to the flowers and lawn. For the most part, the things we discussed were trivial, and that in itself was part of the bonding. Of course, at times we discussed major professional decisions or world crises, but what ties a couple together, I think, are the insignificant details of daily life—the natural weaving of the fabric of our lives.

The loss of that sharing has been inexplicably painful to me. I have never been able to explain this loss to friends satisfactorily. Kee no longer ventures a comment about anything, nor is her occasional response reassuring, for, while I can't know definitively, I doubt whether she follows much of what I say. Silence now dominates this time of the early evening. The voicing of our concerns and experiences was so basic to our shared life that its absence reminds me of a sparkling, life-giving spring that has entirely dried up.

Let me give you an example of our sharing before the coming of Alzheimer's. One evening, when we sat down on the patio, I wanted to talk about a TV production of the previous night. Actually, I had wanted to talk about it then, but Kee often deflected discussion until she had more time to respond. I was always ready to babble away immediately after a movie, play, or concert. She preferred distancing herself from the experience.

On that particular evening I asked, "Have you had time to think about *Billy Budd* yet? Can we talk about it now?" The production was part of the Armstrong Circle Theater series we had seen the previous night. I thought it enthralling, brilliantly acted, superbly cast, genuinely moving. When it ended, we both moved instinctively to cut off the television. Neither of us wanted the experience to be spoiled by commercials or the sitcom coming up next. Stopping the television was like leaving the theater and going to the nearest coffee shop. I wanted to voice my responses, sift through the many strengths and the few weaknesses of the production, to come to some intellectual conclusion about the performance and about the issues Melville posed. Kee, always the more insightful one, didn't want to talk at all.

Twenty-two hours later, after a long day's work, she was ready to discuss our shared experience. We had few disagreements about the production. She, too, thought it splendidly done. After talking about the performances of the actors and the casting, I moved to the moral and ethical issues Melville posed and his resolution. I wanted to know what Kee thought about Vere's decision to execute Budd. For her, that was too intellectual a question, too rarefied. What she stressed was the need to identify with the feelings of all the characters, to feel the pain and confusion of the sailors and particularly the responsibility weighing on Captain Vere as he tried to balance his personal feelings against the discipline required of his office. She was even more in touch with the bitter, sadistic qualities of Claggert than I was.

By focusing so heavily on an intellectual analysis of the play, I was losing some of what makes a good play so germane to our lives. On the stage or in a film we watch actors portraying people with whom we must identify at an emotional level. Understanding is a function of melding intelligence and feelings. We are, in fact, less likely to be changed by the rational than by the emotional.

As we talked, arguing creatively, jostling one another for position, we agreed on the necessity of thoughtful consideration and response. Kee wasn't denying the importance of mind. Rather, she was forcing me to consider the whole person. When I wanted to chatter away, she wanted time to get in touch with her feelings about what she had witnessed.

Wait! I just realized something. That conversation couldn't have occurred on our patio. The production I'm talking about was back in the late fifties or early sixties when we were living in a different house. We didn't have a patio. We probably were sitting on a screened-in back porch. It's odd that my memory transferred the time to a more recent period. I'm certain that we had a conversation about *Billy Budd,* and I'm equally certain that our sharing of insights helped reshape my understanding of the play. My memory maintained a truth but reset the occasion. Kee's memory has retained neither conversation nor location. How different are we, really? Certainly Kee cannot now carry on the kind of conversation we had forty years ago, but are her feelings any less intense? How much has she changed? How different are we?

As a psychotherapist Kee would not have been surprised that in my first recalling of our conversation I was wrong about where it occurred. She would have focused on what the memory meant to me and why from all the other things we shared, I find this particular episode so . . . well, memorable is the right word.

How do I know Kee was a good therapist? Certainly I had no first-hand experience with her in such a role, but there are other ways to know. Most of her referrals came from physicians and former clients. There was more positive evidence: Kee reading me a note which she received from a former patient in which the appreciation and gratitude of the anonymous writer flowed out; one of my friends telling me that at a party he met someone who proudly claimed Kee as his therapist, praising her insightfulness and ability to probe without controlling; Kee bringing home a bronze plaque that a patient finishing therapy had brought her. The plaque is still on her desk, a desk she has not used in a long, long time. The lines on the plaque are from T. S. Eliot:

>We shall not cease from exploration
>And the end of our exploring
>Will be to arrive where we began
>And know the place for the first time.

Whoever took the time to find those lines, have them engraved, and give them to his therapist was not only appreciative, but also had a good understanding of the process.

The only incident related to her professional skills that I ever directly observed occurred, interestingly enough, in an antique store. Kee was looking at some cut glass. I was some distance away looking at some old volumes. Suddenly the rather sedate atmosphere of the shop was shaken by a loud cry of "Coach." A man of about forty bounded over to her and literally lifted her off her feet in a bear hug. He called out again, "Nancy, come over here and meet Coach." A moment later an attractive woman arrived and was introduced to Kee by her husband. I was close enough to hear the woman say, "You saved our marriage." Like an artist, Kee opened eyes and ears to beauty and helped people sculpt their own lives.

I remember telling one of my sons that it's unfortunate that most of the metaphors extolling success in life are game metaphors in which winning or losing is everything and victory can be demonstrated by a score. Life, I suggested, is an art form. In playing a concerto, a violinist is not trying to win; that's impossible if you are interpreting Beethoven. Rather, the artist is trying to realize an ideal, seeking to fulfill his or her understanding of the composer's creation. No performance is perfect, although it may be brilliant and extraordinarily skillful. Painters and sculptors can never be entirely satisfied with their work, work that is rarely "finished." Kee did not fully succeed in rendering the ideals she envisioned, but she grew in her particular art in experience after experience. Although she left behind no tangible works like compositions or paintings, Kee was, I think, a consummate artist. Then came the ravaging effects of Alzheimer's. Everything is past tense. The artist has gone away.

Lost in these musings, I have not noticed that the sun has half disappeared. There are enough clouds to assure a beautiful sunset. In our earlier housing, sunsets were not important. Walls, fences, other houses obscured their beauty—except in Colorado where there was an unobstructed view and we could wait patiently for the sun to dress the sky in golden hues, oohing and aahing when our ranking of the sunset rose from a four to an eight or nine. I don't remember who first suggested a rating system. With my compulsiveness and need to reduce things to manageable proportions, I probably did. Remarkably, we usually agreed whether a sunset rated above an eight.

In the "Snuggery" we were amazed to find that midwestern sunsets often surpass those of Colorado. From our dining room, we've seen some so astonishing that they smashed the ratings, forcing higher standards for nines and tens. When we mentioned this to a scientist friend, he simply said, "Smog." That's not a pleasant explanation, but it doesn't detract from the sheer beauty of some evenings. When we purchased the condo, I wrote to a friend: "We've found the perfect place for us. It's in the city, which we treasure, slightly above the bustle of the streets, and, even at our age, we can look East as well as West." At the time we didn't realize how much time would be spent looking to the west, to sunsets, to the end of a day, to our own demise.

Most of the sun is now covered by a cloud with gilded edges. It is the kind of beauty that has to be experienced. Like a rainbow, it can't be captured in photographs, paintings, or words. Friends in an apartment above us share our fascination and awe. Sometimes the phone will ring, and an excited voice will say, "Look, look, it might be a ten!" Or we might call them and say, "Drop what you're doing. Run to the window. It's glorious."

When there are few clouds, the view is merely awesome. The power of the sun is always there. Other evenings, as cumulus clouds gather on the horizon, the sky takes on colors in which golds blend with blues. Slashes of crimson and garnet sweep across the sky. Long lines of blue and gray suggest a variety of purples merging toward black. The scene is one of prodigal beauty, colors rampant on a limitless canvas. Then it is gone, swiftly sometimes, lingering in paler tones at other times, but gone, leaving only the memory and the excitement.

In the months of May and October, the sun sets behind the bell tower of the seminary west of our apartment. The sky seems to take on added luster. The sun seen through the aperture of the tower suggests a penetrating eye.

On this evening, although I wouldn't rank the sunset higher than a seven, I'm not disappointed. Pastels sometimes fit one's mood better than garish oils. The rosy hue with the light blue background turning darker and darker is pleasing. I take Kee's hand, saying nothing.

After Kee has several cigarettes and drinks her water, I fix our drinks—a tablespoon of scotch in water for her, a Manhattan for myself. The Manhattan before dinner is a delightful self-indulgence. Whether it improves my digestion is irrelevant. Nursing a drink slowly before preparing supper, swirling the ice, entranced by the deep shade of amber, watching the cherry nestled against the bottom; it's a ritual. I allow myself only one, although there are certainly times when I want to get sloshed, to bemoan my loneliness, but I know I have to guard against too much booze and, equally important, against feelings of self-pity.

In a kitchen cabinet there are a number of cut glass tumblers that Kee purchased in antique shops over many years. At one time we had twenty or thirty. Some were dropped, some given away, but we still have ten or twelve. I choose two, studying the intricate patterns of the glass and wondering where she found these two. They could have come from any state between Colorado and the East Coast. At one time Kee could have told me where she bought them, for each glass in the collection is distinctive, and she had a great memory for such purchases.

In antique shops Kee was browser, appraiser, and student. If the shop owner knew some area of antiques well, Kee was adept at discovering that specialty and learning from the dealer. Her enthusiasm and appreciation for almost any well-crafted object quickly won approval and honest advice from reputable dealers. As for me, twenty minutes in an antique shop was about as much as I could take. When we vacationed together, while she was investigating shops, I was either on a golf course or engrossed in one of the books I always carried to see me through what I knew would be several tedious hours. Not one of her glasses was a rash purchase. They were carefully, thoughtfully considered and lovingly, individually selected.

Now what dealers call the "provenance" of each glass is lost. Perhaps some day a great-grandchild might be told that the glasses belonged to their great-grandmother, Ya-Ya, and old Grumps. I rather like the thought and set the glasses down carefully. I mustn't break glasses with such promising futures.

As we sit together at the table, sipping our drinks—well, I sip, Kee tends to take long draws on her straw, consuming the watered Scotch too rapidly—I think about what I need to do to get supper ready. Some of our friends marvel at the fact that I've cooked nearly every meal for the past eight years, the only exceptions being those occasions when a friend brought food in or when one of our children was at home and cooked dinner. I don't find my cooking extraordinary. If one likes to eat well, and accordingly detests frozen dinners, if one's spouse is unable to cook, then the only option is learning to do it oneself. No, the time spent cooking has been mostly pleasurable. I'm even trying to elevate my skills from those of a crude craftsman to those of an artist. I don't even mind shopping about twice a week.

What I do detest is planning weekly menus. When Kee's dementia was first diagnosed, she was able to make suggestions and indicate preferences. Now if I were to ask her what she wanted, she would not be able to answer so general a question. A more specific question like "Would you prefer chicken or fish tonight?" might produce a response, even "I don't know." That's a perfectly rational response, isn't it?

Once I became accustomed to the fact that I was entirely on my own, I attempted to plan weekly menus around three principles: nutritional balance, what I remembered enjoying the last time I prepared it, and boredom. Because there are only a few things that Kee won't eat, I have a relatively free hand. Unfortunately I've also discovered that even if you have twenty-five ways to prepare chicken, chicken is still chicken, and soon becomes boring.

As the months turned into years, my difficulties with menu selection became increasingly acute. If I sat down at the table with pen and paper and a box of coupons and asked, "What shall we eat this week?" I not only drew a blank but became antagonistic to the whole process.

Finally I found a partial solution to the problem of too much choice and too little information. I developed a file of some fifty recipes— from macaroni and cheese to lamb à la pesto, from hamburgers to Venetian chicken. There are Greek, French, Italian, Oriental, and German recipes in addition to old American standards like beef stew and pot roast. From this file I now randomly draw six cards each week. If I draw a recipe I know I don't want to prepare or eat, I return the card and draw another. Or one recipe might remind me of a dish I do want, and I then switch to that. I draw only six cards because once a week I fix steak, Kee's favorite meal.

The beauty of my system is that the initial stage, the drawing of six cards, now has a magical element to it. By ignoring probability theory, I can feel that I am being directed to prepare beef stroganoff if I draw that card. Yet if we had beef stroganoff the previous week, and I'm tired of it, I can exercise free will, return that menu to the file case and feel equally chosen to cook chicken and pasta with an alfredo sauce.

Tonight's menu says pork chops. I drew the card for veal chops, but at the time decided that I wanted some good, old-fashioned, greasy Southern pork chops. The decision probably rested upon a sense that I needed a reward for having followed a sensible diet for several weeks in a row—fish, chicken, lots of green salads and fruits, the things that nutritional experts encourage. Now I shall indulge in forbidden fruit.

One concession to my Southern childhood is the small jar of bacon drippings I keep. Pork chops, dusted with flour and seasoned salt and pepper, fried in bacon grease. Just the right thing to increase my cholesterol level. But I'll also cook some vegetables, omit potatoes with butter, and make a salad using vinegar and just a tad of olive oil—well, maybe put on some blue cheese crumbles. The crumbles will regrettably offset the sacrifice of the potatoes traded for the bacon grease; nevertheless, we will have blue cheese crumbles. Kee likes them very much.

I light another cigarette for her and explain that I'll be in the kitchen for a while but will check every now and then to see if she needs anything. I don't think she understands what I'm saying, but she seems reassured. In the kitchen my first step is to take the salad vegetables from the refrigerator, put them in the sink with water and pour ice over them to get everything crisp. Kee taught me that. And she also purchased a spinner to dry the vegetables once they are crisp. I then put the flour and spices into a small plastic bag, put the bacon grease on to heat, dip the chops in milk, and toss the chops in the bag to coat them. While the chops are cooking (and the grease spattering), I pull down a small saucepan, put a quarter cup water in it, and take a full cup of frozen vegetables from the freezer. By the time I've turned the chops, the vegetables are done.

There are several leftover cornsticks I made three days ago, which, I decide, will make this a truly Southern dinner, even if I'm not preparing turnip greens. The important thing is to remember to take the cornbread out of the oven before reducing the "sticks" to charcoal. By the time the chops are well done, reassuringly browned with just enough charring on the edge to enhance the grease and cholesterol, I've made and tossed the salad and warmed the bread.

Meals have always been central to our life. As a family we always shared breakfast and dinner. When I was a child, family meals were taken for granted. I assumed that all families sat down together to eat breakfast and the evening meal. When Kee and I married, we carved out time in the day to eat those meals together and succeeded in maintaining the tradition until our children went off to college. Sometimes anger from perceived slights or misunderstandings spilled out, but frequently there was good conversation to be shared. Our children reported how other families grabbed bits of food on the run and ate together only on holidays. Occasionally they even admitted liking our habit of eating together.

I particularly remember certain meals alone with Kee, some of them celebrating birthdays or anniversaries, some in public places, some private, meals when there was sharing, literally and symbolically. Food was transformed into energy, and separateness was momentarily transformed into oneness as we shared thoughts about our children and their plans and our hopes for one another and our future.

With the ravages of AD, full sharing and oneness disappeared, and eating out together with pleasure became impossible. I can't recall all the details of where and when, but Kee began to talk less. When she did talk, it was often about something from the distant past that disturbed her. She became clumsy, spilling food, turning over glasses. Getting her to the bathroom in time became first an ordeal and finally an impossibility.

As her incontinence became extreme, we stopped going out to eat, even to our neighborhood bar and grill. Table conversation metamorphosed into my monologues and her confused, often unfathomable, and always brief utterances. Gradually there was no conversation, only a pretense of listening. I was distressingly slow to recognize what was happening, or was I simply unwilling to understand? Then with her falls and regression to a near-childlike state, I needed to feed her, to coax her to eat, to plead that she eat vegetables or salads.

The history of our relationship over the last eight years can be summarized by what has happened at meals. In fact, if we had recorded our meals over the fifty-plus years of our intimacy, we could follow our relationship in capsule form. There were the early picnics and outdoor grills, she diminutive and simply dressed but radiant, myself tall, thin, faking a maturity I did not possess. There were church-sponsored lobster dinners in New England; evenings when friends joined us for meatloaf, hot dogs, or braised beef short ribs as we struggled to make ends meet. Then came those meals when mopping up spills and coaxing our children to eat caused us to forget what we were eating. There were Thanksgiving dinners for friends from other countries. Later, as our financial situation improved, there were special occasions when we went out to fancy, upscale restaurants for anniversaries and birthdays. Neither of us liked fast-food places. When we were poor, we simply didn't eat out often, saving what we could for an annual splurge on our anniversary. Food, food carefully, lovingly prepared, gracefully served on china, with white tablecloths, flowers, and quiet music. We were, I suppose, suckers for atmosphere and delicious food! Remembering great restaurants in Chicago, San Francisco, Atlanta, New Orleans, New York, Denver, and Washington still causes me to salivate. A few were so extravagantly expensive that we could not really enjoy our meals, but most provided immediate gratification. The memories will continue even as the details become increasingly jumbled.

One oddity is the fact that some of our most ferocious arguments occurred when we ate out alone. Neither of us liked to argue when the children were present so the more turbulent disagreements developed when we were dining at moderately priced restaurants, never at the most expensive ones. In that, at least, we were prudent— don't ruin an expensive evening.

Once I've finished the chops, have the meal on the table, and sit down to feed Kee, I begin to think about the cornbread I did not burn. Frequently I forget to rescue bread from the oven before it is cremated. In recent months, when I've invited friends in for dinner, on three consecutive occasions we were halfway through dinner before I remembered the bread. Twice it smoked up the kitchen, once setting off the fire alarm.

In each instance our friends politely insisted that bread was not necessary. Their insistence was more strident the night the fire alarm began blaring. Nevertheless, it irritates me that I can prepare a full three- or four-course meal and still not remember the bread. After the first failure, I made a detailed list of things to do and when to do them —and still forgot the bread. There's something alarmingly symptomatic about this pattern. Why do I burn bread? The obvious answer is that I try to do too much. But I don't like that excuse. It relegates what some of our friends call my "heroism" in carrying on to a condition closer to comedy.

Another possibility is what our guests suggest. The bread is incidental to the meal, not of primary importance, and therefore it just slips my mind. But the possibility that really disturbs and intrigues me is the symbolic meaning—bread as the staff of life. "Let us break bread together" implores the old spiritual I learned as a teenager. Do you think it's possible that something in my brain short-circuits when it comes to serving bread? I can remember to put it in the oven, so it's not a question of intent. Why can't I remember to take it out? Maybe subconsciously I'm declaring that my staff of life is gone, although she sits at the table smiling. She can no longer help me prepare dinner; she can no longer help me to remember to put out napkins (which I also often forget); she can no longer help me remember to take the bread out of the oven before it burns. Am I burning the bread in repressed protest?

Or could there be something more deliberate working in my mind—a will to sabotage? Could some portion of me be declaring: you pretend to have everything under control, to be master of the kitchen, to be master of life and time. Admit that you are basically incapable of coping skillfully in the kitchen. Let's see what you do with this incinerated bread.

Throughout this silent cross-examination (sorry, another bad pun), I continue to feed Kee—a bit of chop, of vegetables, a sip of tea, repeat. I try to attend to my food, to dismiss my bizarre thoughts about not successfully serving bread, but I can't let the concern go. Slowly, a memory takes shape, materializing like an actor's image in *Star Wars*. Kee is in our kitchen, kneading dough on a bread board. On a shelf nearby, a bowl holds another batch of bread which has been set aside to rise. Kee's face is radiant with pleasure. A long-forgotten conversation gradually slips into focus. The children and I are eating slices of delicious bread fresh from the oven. I ask Kee if baking bread is worth the trouble when she has so much to do. She smiles and says, "It's the most creative thing I do. It's almost like giving birth. The feel of the dough as I knead it is like working with clay in a potter's studio."

Somewhere in a kitchen cabinet there is still a small file box containing her bread recipes: French bread, cholla, rye salt flutes, cheese bread, Russian black bread, Swedish limpa, popovers, and many others I can't remember, but each distinctive, each unlike anything I make or even that I can buy from a bakery. Kee had no dough mixer, no special oven, just two desires: to identify creatively with an action shared by others century after century and to give her family the best she could.

Somehow this memory clarifies why the sharing of bread is so important a symbol for me. It doesn't explain why I continue to burn bread, but it helps me understand why I find my failures so disturbing.

Most of my musings are too convoluted, too ingenuous, and, at times, utterly naive. Why am I so given to looking for meanings, to self-interrogation? At the core of my being I feel like a satellite bombarded by too many radio waves. Only satellites can't feel. When caught up in the demands of my career and, I ruefully admit, too little in the needs of my family, I wasn't plagued by such ruminations. I made decisions and acted on them. If I didn't fully understand the reasons for my actions, I could at least perform them without an excess of misgivings. Now, with my time and thoughts occupied by someone I love, who desperately needs me, I'm confused and self-confusing. I've set a course and followed it, but that does not give me peace of mind or satisfaction.

We finish dinner. The chops are good, not the best I've done, but satisfying. Again I have to leave Kee and return to the kitchen to do the dishes, another chore I don't mind. Rinsing the plates and the pot is no trouble. The frying pan, however, reminds me that all pleasures have their costs.

Like the time after lunch, the hour or so after dinner is dead time. Early in Kee's illness I was able to go into the study and get some work done. For the last several years, that has been impossible. There is the danger that she might burn herself or even start a fire if she were allowed to have cigarettes at her disposal, although by now she is unable to light one. A child-guard lighter baffles her. If she could use the lighter, she might light the filter tip. Those considerations, however, are less important than the way I feel if I leave her alone for more than the few minutes required to do dinner or clean up afterward.

When I am gone more than a few minutes, I return to find her head lolling on her breast. When she looks up her eyes register distress, perhaps even fear. I would prefer an angry "Where have you been?" to this silent condemnation. Guilt is never far away in my current relationship with Kee, and it's a guilt I can neither account for nor resolve. Day after day I ask myself whether I am doing all that I can for her. Did I give up too soon trying to find a miraculous cure? Is there some as yet unknown herb in a South American rain forest I might find? What if it really isn't Alzheimer's? Should I seek other diagnoses? It was probably guilt that led me to delay so long in getting professional caregivers to relieve me during the day. I no longer feel guilty leaving her with such support, and she has come to accept my absence without visible signs of distress. Without that relief I think I would have become useless to her as well as to myself, a physical and psychological derelict.

At night, however, when we are at home alone, I still find that guilt imprisons me. I might try to go into another room for a brief time, but I can't bear the silent condemnation on my return. Or am I imagining that censure? I don't know and can't know. Perhaps she is only confused. But if I have contributed to that, then I have partially failed her. In any event, I must live with my own perceptions.

On nights when Kee gives signs of wanting to go back to bed, and I have tucked her in, I have no qualms about going to the family room or my study because I see no consternation or anger in her eyes. No longer do I tell her I will be back in thirty minutes because time is incomprehensible to her. Usually I say, "I'll be back soon."

There are things I can do at the table with her—write checks or letters, rough out things I need to get done, make out my indispensable lists—anything that does not involve intense concentration. Not only have I given up reading at the table, I've also given up using my laptop in the dining room. Attending to her is incompatible with concentrating on anything else.

During the early years of her illness, we went into the family room about eight o'clock and watched television for several hours. I vividly recall one of the early signs of her dementia. On an evening in mid-December I scanned the television programs, hoping to find a program she would enjoy. There it was—*It's a Wonderful Life*. Over the years we must have watched it a dozen times or more, but we hadn't yet seen it that particular year. I asked her if she would enjoy seeing it again. Her response was "What is it?" I assured her that she remembered Jimmy Stewart struggling with his sense of failure, his bumbling, guardian angel who wanted to earn his wings, the sour, greedy old banker, the grateful citizens of the town, and the little girl saying, "Whenever a bell rings. . . ."

She didn't. Not one character or episode could she recall. Certain that the visual images would spark some recall, I turned on the program. When the dance floor opened and the celebrants plunged into the pool, I said, "I know you remember that scene." She remembered nothing, and soon drifted out of the room because nothing was coherent to her—there was no story line, there was no drama—only baffling images moving about making no sense to her.

That evening was only a few weeks before the diagnosis of Alzheimer's. Recalling that evening, I am troubled by my refusal to face reality. I continued to hope that depression was the cause of her forgetfulness. Tomorrow would be different. I tried to bury the incident away in remote recesses of my mind. I could not avoid, however, a new awareness. I realized that whenever I commented on a television program, her response was general, open-ended. "Wasn't that exciting?" might elicit a "Yes." Or "Look at that beautiful landscape" might trigger "It is beautiful." I might turn to her and say, after some miscellaneous information about tiger cubs, "Did you know that?" And she would respond, "I don't think so." She was possibly playing a role she had chosen. Do not admit the truth. Be courteous, responsive, and he won't know that I can't understand what he's talking about. But that sounds too rational, doesn't it? More likely, she was unaware of her disorientation.

Tonight I rather hope that Kee will want to go lie down. Then I can send some e-mails. I am determined not to spend more time at the dining table. No more solitaire—at least not today. No more scanning of magazines in which I have little interest. Television is a possibility, but I don't want to wheel her into the family room without some sign of acquiescence. On the nights when she lies down right after supper and I get her up after an hour or so, she protests if I attempt to move her from the bedroom to the family room. She has staked out the dining room as her place.

Expecting agreement when I ask, "Do you want to lie down?" I am frustrated by "I don't think so" and decide that I will take her to the family room for television whether or not she agrees. Under stacks of newspapers, I locate the weekly listings. Only three programs seem worthwhile. The first is a documentary dealing with parental participation in public schools. I'm pleased that it's being shown but am in no mood to watch it, and I know that Kee would become restless within minutes. The second is *Mystery!* but the description is familiar. Not only have I seen it before, but I remember the outcome. If it starred one of my favorite sleuths, Inspector Morse or Brother Cadfael, I might watch it again even though it, too, would make Kee restless. When I experience sufficient pleasure, I confess that I find ways to talk her through her restlessness.

The third program features Sherpa guides in Nepal. That interests me because I know now that I will never go to that part of the world. You're smiling. No, you're right. I do not watch sitcoms. (I once watched fifteen minutes of *Seinfeld* to see what the hoopla was about.) No, I don't object to them. Maybe I'm afraid I would become addicted.

Trying to decide whether I will watch the travelogue on Nepal, I remember that for some time I've wanted to rewatch our own travel tapes of trips made between 1985 and 1994. Four years or so have passed since I looked at any of them. Possibly, by studying them closely, I might pick up clues as to when Kee's dementia should have been evident to me. That I ignored the early signs, or simply failed to recognize that there were signs, troubles me for reasons I can't explain. Was I so inattentive to her? Was I so preoccupied with other matters that I never saw signs that must have been there? The children agree that there were clear indications of problems by 1992, but before then? Maybe in the images I can find clues for which memory is insufficient or false.

Our travels before 1994 are recorded on slides I transferred to VCR tape by using our camcorder, not purchased until late 1994, to film slides I projected onto the wall. I then copied the camcorder's eight-millimeter cassette onto the VCR tape. A professional firm would have produced higher quality tapes, but when I made them I was looking for the cheapest way. Anyway, I enjoyed going through the old slides with Kee and, with camcorder sound, was able to comment on where the pictures were taken and what the circumstances were. In 1995, although Kee's dementia had been confirmed, she was able to watch with me and seemed to follow what I was doing with interest.

Four tapes might tell me something. The first is principally a collection of slides made in Colorado in the mid-eighties; the second from a visit to Spain we made shortly after our daughter's wedding in 1990. A third consists of slides taken in England in 1992, by which time my children and I had become very concerned about Kee's depression, her drinking, and her lack of stamina. The last tape consists of slides made in Greece in 1993—before the diagnosis of the dementia, but well past the time when we feared mental illness.

Convinced that I know how I want to spend the evening, rather than pose a question I say, enthusiastically, "Let's watch the tapes of our travels!" I watch Kee closely, hoping to see a glimmer of recognition, a desire to go back to view times that have slipped away from her. No such signs are evident, but she responds "O.K.," which is enough. I wheel her into the family room, setting her up again at the small table where she can smoke and where I can place a glass of water for her.

The slides of Colorado tell me nothing. Most are scenic shots of rock formations, sunsets, distant panoramas. The few slides in which Kee appears were taken around the campsite. In one she is reading at a table I fashioned for her out of juniper and two-by-fours. In another she is doing something at the stove in our dining tent. At least there is evidence that she was reading and cooking as late as 1987. I can tell nothing from her expressions except that she seems happy and content. I remember, however, how short of breath she was in the first few days of our summer visits, but that is true of most people at nine thousand feet. Next tape.

The slides of Spain three years later don't reveal much either, but they jar my memory. We went to Spain because a dear friend had inherited a casa on the Costa del Sol and invited us to use it for three weeks. We jumped at the chance, for, apart from travel and a few other expenses, the cost would be negligible. By Spanish law, our friend was required to retain a housekeeper and gardener until the house was sold. Even our meals would be prepared. Turning down such an opportunity was inconceivable. We went.

Much of the time we stayed near the casa, only a few hundred yards from the Mediterranean, but we did take five days to go to Seville, Cordoba, and Granada. The slides in which Kee appears are scenic—she is looking out over the gardens in Granada, gazing at the cathedral in Seville, or wandering through side streets of Cordoba as we sought the home of Maimonides. Only one slide provides any clue. It is a picture I made just before we left for Madrid. Kee is posing with the young couple who served as gardener and housekeeper. She is smiling broadly. Both of them have their arms around her. Her broad-brimmed hat casts shadows on the young man.

The clue is the shadows. Apart from the trip to the cities of Andalusia, she would not go out of the house except to sit on the patio in the late evening. It was too hot, always too hot. She was right about that. August is *not* the ideal time to visit southern Spain. Only once did I get her to go on a brief day trip—a short drive to Ronda to see the bullring and the deep chasm dividing the old city from the new. The heat was tolerable in the morning and even through lunch at an outdoor cafe where there was a spectacular view of the chasm cut by the river over thousands of years. It being the dry season, the river was reduced to stagnant pools.

In the Michelin guide I had read of prehistoric drawings in a cave just a few miles north of Ronda. Kee did not want to go, but I convinced her that we would never be back. Perhaps she gave in just because she didn't want to disappoint me. By the time we reached the caves, the heat was oppressive. As we climbed up a mountain to the entry of the cave, Kee almost collapsed. I half carried her the rest of the way, assuring her that the cave would be cool. It was even chilly, but she showed virtually no interest in the primitive drawings of deer, of fish, and of a pregnant horse. Nor did the signs of ancient camp fires interest her.

Her lack of interest in things that at one time would have excited her surely revealed something. That she was incapable of dealing with the heat may not signify anything, but the lethargy that prevailed throughout the trip, her indifference to virtually everything, continued to confuse and irritate me. She did, however, enjoy our late evening meals prepared by the young Spanish woman, a superb cook whose *paella* was the best we ate in Spain, and served on the patio. Both the woman and her husband were extraordinarily attentive to Kee. They obtained fresh figs from the market every morning for her breakfast—*higos* if I remember correctly. The figs were large, firm, delicious—the best we had ever eaten. Were the two servants, who did not understand English, better readers of her attitude and body language than I was? What might they have told me if I had understood more than a few Spanish phrases?

In 1990, when we made the trip, I alternated between concern for her and annoyance that she was squandering our unique opportunity. I made some effort to learn very basic Spanish; she made none. I reread *The Sun Also Rises*, Hotchner's *Iberia*, Jan Morris's book on Andalusia and other travel books; Kee read nothing before or during the trip. We were only a few hundred yards from the beach, and in the evenings, with the sun below the horizon, the stroll was alluringly romantic; she never accompanied me despite my pleadings. Once in a while she made half-hearted efforts to play backgammon with me. What she did like was my complete attention. At times that, too, was annoying, particularly when I wanted to stroll the streets of the town and sit in outdoor cafes. Retrospectively I can admit that I was annoyed mostly because she was putting a damper on my pleasure.

Somewhere, in one of our closets is a journal I kept while in Spain. That might tell me more than the slides. Likely, however, the entries will reveal more about my delight with Spanish culture and the architecture and paintings we saw than any significant perspective on Kee. The journal is probably a monument to blindness and insensitivity. I was looking only at symptoms—symptoms that I thought confirmed her depression. Not once did it occur to me that the symptoms were overt signals of the approaching shadow of Alzheimer's.

Sitting before the television, in a rocker which belonged to my father, I think about what the slides did not reveal. As I watched the Spanish slides and thought of shadows, I thought of the word *men-*

ace. My associations with the word intrigue me. Is its root in any way related to "dementia?" Perhaps they have some common etymology. I think of scurrying off to the dictionary to see if the two words are related. I've always thought of something menacing as an object, force, or person outside myself. Is it possible that anything seen as *menacing* might be more an internalized fear than an external phenomenon? Well, the matter intrigues me but not enough to make me climb out of my chair. Maybe some other time. Anyway, they ought to be related. I'm sure that in Kee's mind in the early nineties, nothing was more menacing than her fears that she was slipping into dementia. And she couldn't tell me! Was it my fault, or could she not admit it to herself?

Removing the tape on Spain, I insert the one on England from 1992. Once again, the slides reveal little. There are seven or eight in which she is looking at the camera. In two she stands with a friend before some fifteenth-century ruins. We went there for lunch from Dartmouth where the friend lives. In one Kee is smiling, but the smile is not the gracious, enchanting smile of earlier years. It seems forced, and her eyes betray awareness that she is posing. In the other, although our friend is smiling broadly, Kee is not. Her face looks haggard, drawn, her eyes unfocused.

Since I've frequently been captured in a snapshot looking like a half-wit with mouth half open and eyes three-quarters closed, I gave her appearance in this slide little thought when we first looked at it. I said something like: "This is awful of you, but it's the best picture we have of Patty. Shall we keep it?" I can't recall her response. Did she respond, or did I merely *think* then that she was observing with interest? I wonder if, in that fall of 1992 when we got the slides back from the developer, she responded, "whatever" or "I guess so." I have no idea. By 1994 she was adept at giving our friends the illusion that she understood them when I knew she didn't. Had she practiced on me earlier?

We all throw up defenses at times. Early in childhood I instinctively realized that you can pretend to be actively engaged in a discussion or pretend to be attentive to a reprimand. All that is needed is the proper countenance—a smile or frown or look of regret—and occasional eye contact. People want to be understood so badly that they assume understanding where there may be little or none. In the classroom I have called on a student who seemed deeply involved with what we were doing and then watched that attentive look dissolve into utter confusion. The student's mind was off in some distant world.

Kee must have learned this "social grace" early in life, too, and perhaps she carried it over when she found herself in the tangled swamps of Alzheimer's disease. I am inclined to think that she never quite realized what was happening. I should have been more alert, more perceptive, and less self-deceiving. My deep concern for her and our relationship caused me to refuse to acknowledge that her deterioration was beyond her control. For the present, I want to avoid entering a plea. I cannot acquit myself, but "guilty" seems too harsh a judgment.

The Greek slides from 1993 remain to offer some relief from the terrible and unanswerable questions I pose. In Spain and in England, we traveled as cheaply as we could, relying on the hospitality of friends, staying in B and B's, avoiding expensive restaurants. For our trip to Greece, we decided to fund the trip with some money from Kee's retirement accounts. We had been fortunate in our earnings and relatively thrifty in our spending. Propelled by a desire to travel, we built savings accounts. Assuming that our daily costs in retirement could be met from my retirement funds, we planned to use Kee's savings for travel. By 1993 she had been retired for almost three years. Over that time, her retirement accounts grew beyond expectations. It was time to begin traveling slightly above "steerage" class. I also reasoned that since Kee was not physically strong, it was important to make the trip easy for her. Perhaps the trip to Greece would shake her out of her listless, depressive state.

Kee showed little interest in planning the details of the trip, but by then I was not surprised. I suggested that we begin the trip, after a day of rest from the long flight, with a cruise of the Cyclades on a small, inexpensive vessel that carried only thirty people. Then we would attempt the more arduous part of our visit, a bus trip through the Peloponnesus, on to Delphi, and back to Athens. Before flying home we could take a larger ship to see Istanbul, Ephesus, Rhodes, Patmos, and Crete. She agreed amiably to everything I suggested. The cruises were my way of avoiding the jumping from hotel to hotel she found so exhausting. She didn't read any of the literature I gave her, but although I was annoyed, I did not see that as cause to cancel the trip.

Now reviewing the slides, slides that recall memories of details that had slipped into cracks, I think the entire trip was for my benefit. Although a trip to Greece was something she had wanted to do for years, by 1993 she may not really have wanted to attempt it. She may have agreed to everything and indicated a willingness to go only because I wanted to go. On the small yacht, we frequently sat together on deck, but only after constant urging could I get her to go into the villages where we docked. Usually gregarious, she made little attempt to relate to other passengers. Yes, she smiled cordially, occasionally agreeing with what was said, but as I recall now, she contributed to conversation only when I asked her to narrate a story about our children or about her days running the preschool center in the housing project. She didn't even respond angrily to outrageously prejudiced comments from some of our fellow passengers. There was a time when she would have quickly challenged them.

On the bus trip through the Peloponnesus, Kee developed a terrible migraine headache that lasted for three of the five days we traveled. When she could not be in a hotel room, she simply stayed on the bus. By the time we reached Delphi, I was no longer annoyed but deeply concerned. Clearly she was ill. The headache exacerbated her condition, but I knew it was not the only cause. Something worse than depression was involved. At times she did not know or care where we were. She only wanted to go home to our Snuggery.

In one slide she is sitting down, crouched in the little shade available. She is wearing sunglasses and the floppy sun hat we bought in England the previous year. Behind her are the ruins of a wall. I well remember where the picture was taken. Even if memory failed me, the adjacent slides declare "the glory of old Greece." She is on the Acropolis within thirty feet of the Parthenon. Were she looking to her right, she would be seeing its massive, elegant columns; glancing to her left she would see the Areopagus where Paul preached. Straight before her she would have seen the stunning figures serving as supporting columns of the Erechtheum. From the tilt of her head, I know that she is attending to none of these wonders. Twenty-three-hundred-year-old ruins are as nothing. Her head is bowed, but not in prayer. She is there and not there, slipping away from present and past, aware only that she is dreadfully uncomfortable. Her response to a question I asked a few minutes after taking this slide still rings in my mind:

"Are you all right?"

"Let's go home." I had brought her there. I had brought her there with money she earned and saved.

It's curious, but for that I do not feel guilty. Stupid, yes! What baffles me is how I pushed so much evidence of her condition into the further corners of my brain. She wanted to make the trip, and if it was only for me, I will not mock her generosity. Or am I only assuming that she wanted to make the trip? I'll never know her motives, but I think she still had sufficient awareness so that there were motives, motives governed by love and sharing. At the time, I thanked her for making the trip possible. We could not have made the trip on my income. I credited her accomplishments and praised her for all of her contributions. I don't feel mortified because I was greedy or lacking in appreciation of all that Kee managed to achieve, but I am mortified by my blindness and inability to see what was developing. I did not understand. I don't understand now either. Then I had to do the best that I could with incomplete understanding. That same situation confronts me now. I can either quit or go on fully knowing how little I comprehend.

Putting the tapes away, I notice tapes of slides taken years earlier on trips we made when Kee was young and healthy. Shortly before our children entered the uncontrollable midteens (Kee was thirty-nine), with a loan from Kee's mother we purchased a tent-trailer from Sears Roebuck for less than five hundred dollars. For the first time we both took extended vacations and set off to see the West. We followed the Platte River through Nebraska, peered into Devil's Canyon in Wyoming, climbed in the Grand Tetons, were chased out of our dining tent by bears in Yellowstone, and caught trout in a river. In California we rode horses on the beach and went to Disneyland. We stood in awe before the White Throne of Zion Canyon. At the Grand Canyon we took a sick child to the clinic and teetered on the edge of the Canyon awestruck by the vastness and the richness of its colors. At Mesa Verde we climbed through the cliff dwellings of a people long vanished. Our investment in the trailer saved us thousands of dollars and gave us indelible memories.

Kee was central to it all. She did most of the cooking and resolved most of the disputes which erupt when three adults (Kee's mother was with us) and three children (ages nine, twelve, and fourteen) inhabit the same space hour after hour. My primary contribution, other than driving the station wagon and packing and unpacking the tent-trailer, came in a burst of inspiration. On the third day out, somewhere near Scott's Bluff, I was beginning to boil over from the children's bickering and complaining. With Solomonic wisdom, I blurted out: "Enough! I don't want to hear one more complaint. Today is

Sunday—no more complaints. Tomorrow Kristin can complain, but no one else. Tuesday, Geoffrey gets to complain, no one else. On Wednesday, Paul, Grandmother on Thursday, Mom on Friday. I get to complain on Saturday. No one can complain if it's not their day. On Sunday, only God can complain!" Miraculously it worked. Kee made it work by converting it into a game. An untimely complaint brought five people down on the unfortunate complainer. Failure to remember that it was your day to complain brought suppressed snickers from five others over wasted opportunity.

I don't even need to look at the slides to remember that trip. We viewed the slides so often as a family that we all remember the exact sequence. Memories, visions, were etched on our minds as vividly as on film and will be retained longer. Our tales of adventures grow more expansive with each viewing. But I'm forgetting—Kee no longer remembers any of it. Or does she? As she sits silently with her head down, I would like to believe that she is rerunning the tape with pleasure. I can't.

The marvels of travel, of sightseeing—the marvels of pictures which trigger memories one never wants to lose. The inconveniences and the weariness of traveling vanish before the pleasure of remembrance. Yet I sometimes worry that our travel fetish is destructive to those places we want to see. On the Acropolis we saw signs imploring people like ourselves not to take stones or bits of marble, yet fellow tourists casually slipped pieces into travel bags for their gardens in Hartford or Hamburg. I've read that the Grand Canyon is suffering environmental shock from the sheer number of visitors. Mount Everest is becoming littered. Even the moon has debris left by astronauts! Some of the grand waterways of the world are despoiled more by tourist vessels and pleasure boats than by commercial ships. I can't help but wonder if it would be better if we all stayed home and watched tapes made by master photographers. But I'm afraid I'm being hypocritical. Offer me free tickets to Italy, and I'll be off immediately! No, that's impossible, but I would go if I could.

I suppose my hypocrisy doesn't trouble me much. Hypocrisy is, I fear, fundamental to human nature.

The ashtray tells me how late it is. While I was watching the travel slides, Kee smoked seven cigarettes. I no longer try to contain her smoking, attending only to the danger of her burning herself. While she smokes, I chew on a pipe, only occasionally lighting it. Kee's glass is empty, and she looks tired, but not once has she complained. Several times she responded to comments I made, but only with stock phrases, "Yes" or "I think so." Has she pretended to be interested? Has she remembered some of our times together? Or is she in some small theater of her own?

When Kee first entered the current phase of Alzheimer's, at times I asked her what she was thinking. It seems impossible to me that her brain is in a comalike state, that she is staring at a blank and silent screen. When I speak, she often appears startled and never gives me any inkling that she is thinking anything. She might smile at me, or she might simply look puzzled. I desperately want to connect with whatever her mind is doing—and can't.

It's too late to catch the local evening news. Turning off the VCR, I switch to *Headline News,* but then decide that Kee needs a change of setting before going to bed. Off goes the television. I roll her back into the dining room and give her another small drink and her evening pills—two Tylenol PM's and a Trazadone. I pour myself a glass of apple juice, smear peanut butter over two crackers, and take two ibuprofen. Perhaps the pills are unnecessary. My leg hasn't bothered me much today. Clearly exercise is making it stronger. I just have to avoid reinjuring my back.

As we sit at the table, I talk about the slides we, or I, watched. For persons of modest means, we have been many places and seen a great deal. Our life together has been full, and I am grateful to Kee, particularly for her steadfastness and encouragement until the dementia brought us crashing to earth. The dreams we once shared—

building a cottage in Colorado, several more trips abroad, especially to Italy—will never be realized, but so much warmth and sharing have been ours that fantasizing about what might have been is foolish.

This slack time of the evening, now a brief period just before putting her to bed, was at one time devoted to cribbage or backgammon. Early in our marriage I tried to interest her in chess. Unfortunately chess too readily revealed basic differences in our personalities. I was aggressive, constantly attacking. She was much more conservative, huddling her forces in defensive postures, always responding to my moves rather than developing an attack strategy of her own. You can understand why we gave up the game. Cribbage and backgammon, on the other hand, are less dependent on strategy. Soon after her earliest clinical symptoms became evident, the counting basic to cribbage began to confuse her. We continued for a while to play backgammon. Perhaps the necessity of moving her men to the limited options the dice dictated made the game simpler, but for a year or so she took pleasure in our play.

Now we are reduced to sitting quietly at the table listening to the classical music station. How much she hears, I cannot know, but her body language says that she is more at ease with a Dvorak concerto or a Bach fugue than with any contemporary pop music. I've also noticed that the few movies, either rented or on television, that seem to give her some pleasure are the "classical" musicals. *My Fair Lady, Fiddler on the Roof,* and *Sound of Music* seem to soothe her, although she does not watch the screen.

I ask Kee if she is ready to go to bed. She nods emphatically. The only difficulty with getting her to bed is moving her from the wheelchair to the bed. Early in the day, she is strong enough to assist. At night, however, her legs are completely limp. To protect my back, I have to move her slowly, shuffling my feet an inch or two at a time to keep her weight squarely in front of me. The several injuries to my back resulted from losing my balance and letting her weight turn me in such a way that my decaying discs pinched the nerves energizing my left leg. Changing her slip-ons at night is also more difficult because of the way I have to bend over the bed.

Once Kee is settled in bed, I put a drop of Xalatan in each of her eyes. The drops have lessened the pressure in each eye so that the ophthalmologist is now less concerned about glaucoma. What will I do if the doctor ever suggests surgery? Would it be worth it to her? She uses her eyes so little now. Or would the obstructed vision that goes with glaucoma cause her further suffering, even panic? And how can I know?

I smooth the sheet over her, kiss her, and perform an Eskimo nose rub, saying, "I'll be along soon." "Promise?" she asks. I promise. Cutting off the light reminds me that her days are limited, probably more than mine. When she was diagnosed with AD the doctor said, "She probably has eight to ten years." I was surprised not only because he was so blunt, but also because my understanding is that no one dies of AD. Later, as I checked the causes of death for Alzheimer's patients, I found that common maladies such as heart disease, pneumonia, cancer, and strokes account for most deaths. AD simply lowers resistance to any illness. Because AD victims often develop difficulties in swallowing and then aspirate food or liquids into their lungs, pneumonia is perhaps the most frequent immediate cause of death. Someday I will likely have to make the decision as to whether I will permit efforts to extend her existence by use of an artificial feeding tube. Already I am talking with the children about those difficult and terrifying options.

So Kee may have only four more years. What if I awaken some morning and find that she died of a stroke during the night? How will I manage? Will I panic? Will I be relieved? I think both reactions inevitable. I have no sense at all of which emotion will be strongest. But this I know, I will miss her dreadfully and know already that for a long time I will flounder about trying to find myself.

I have to go back into the family room to pick up the glasses and empty the ashtray. One wall of that room is covered with family pictures—the children at various ages, Kee and I when we married, our parents, Kee and I in Colorado in camping gear, marriage pictures of two of our children, Kee's sister, our grandparents, and one of Kee's great-grandfather, an itinerant Baptist preacher who continues to look out disapprovingly. In a sense these pictures record who we are and where we have been. Whatever happens, I will want these pictures surrounding me wherever I live.

The living room is a tribute to Kee's decorating skills. Everything has an Oriental theme, the comfortable sofas as well as the uncomfortable Chinese chairs. There are Japanese prints, Chinese paintings, a large French Chinoiserie armoire, antique Chinese chairs, a glass case containing miscellaneous pieces of ivory, a Chinese altar table, a jadeite statuette of a laughing Buddha and one of an old Chinese sage, and lamps made of Chinese vases. Oriental rugs picked up at an auction tie the room together. Each has a story in our life, and the memories, now held only in my mind, will make it difficult for me to dispose of any of them.

This has been our home for more than nine years. Once I lose Kee, will I have a home? We've lived many places. There was the two-room apartment where we lived when we were first married. Then during our first year in graduate school we lived in a two-room attic apartment, a fourth-floor walk-up where the ceiling in both rooms slanted down from a height of eight feet to less than four—the original A-frame, even if it was on the fourth level. With a bed stuck under one side of the bedroom/living room and a small table to eat on squeezed under the wedge of the kitchen, I had to be careful not to strike my head when getting up from either. The only other furniture was a desk and three chairs. If we had friends in, we borrowed more chairs from neighbors on the other side of the stairwell. That's when we were truly poor but happy, unencumbered, adventurous, full of expectations.

Then for two years there was an oddly shaped four-room apartment, part of a three-story building owned by an aged patriarch who even in his eighties ran a grocery store on the ground floor. Designed to suit a plot of land where two streets intersected at odd angles, the apartment didn't have a single square corner. Because each room had an ancient gas jet visible, we assumed the building was constructed before electric lights were readily available. Only later did we discover that Mr. Schevitz, who ran the small grocery, was the original owner and insisted on the gas lines, confident that electric lights were not here to stay. When Mr. Schevitz first showed us the apartment, he beamed, assuring us that there was plenty of room for children. Within months, Kee was pregnant with our first child. Mr. Schevitz could not have been more pleased and daily assured Kee that she was growing ever more beautiful.

When Kee was carrying our second child, we became caretakers of a beach house for two nine-month periods, surviving in the summers by scrambling from one friend's apartment to another's. Married for six years, we had never been in one place for more than two. When I got my first full-time job, we lived in a five-room flat, and there our third child was conceived. After four years we moved into a rented house, then bought our first house—three stories with eight rooms. For the first time our children had separate bedrooms. There for sixteen years we raised our family, entertained friends, and lived comfortably in one place. Then, when our children left, we committed ourselves to a completely illogical move, buying a larger three-story house with twelve spacious rooms. Our justification for the expansion was that Kee's mother would be living with us, and with her would come streams of other relatives for visits of unpredictable lengths. For the first time we had ample space and sufficient funds to do more than makeshift decorating. I think Kee was never happier than when she was choosing antique furnishings for that house.

This is our final residence, our ninth in the fifty-one years we have been married. Will I still be able to call it home when Kee dies? Will I want to stay here? Where is home? If the old sampler saying "home is where the heart is" is correct, then this place will no longer be home. To own a house is not to possess it. With Kee alive, we possessed places. Every room bore her distinctive stamp. Kee had a knack for turning any place we lived into a distinctive expression of ourselves. From the pear crates, planks, and bricks of our early apartments to this living room Kee brought a "touch." Sometimes I thought she was straining our limited funds, but she really had a good sense of what we could and could not afford.

Kee loved auctions, where her "eye" served her well. The things that attracted me she usually vetoed, and in hindsight, I realize she was right. The things that she liked and bought never seemed to transform themselves into horrors. She bought our old four-poster walnut bed in 1977 for seven hundred dollars when pine beds of much poorer quality were selling for two thousand in fashionable furniture stores. Even the uncomfortable Chinese chairs were a "steal." And to be fair, they are more decorative in her scheme than functional.

What makes a house a home is the subject of hundreds of schmaltzy poems as well as old-fashioned samplers, but none of them ever quite expressed my feelings. Such feelings elude definition, lying beyond the province of language. The strange thing is that we nevertheless feel compelled to try to articulate even the vaguest of feelings. It's human nature to spit into the dust of words, trying to make them malleable and cohesive, subject to shaping into a coherent image of what lives in the heart or churns in the gut.

One hundred, two hundred years ago, it was easier to conceptualize and express a concept like home. Before the nineteenth century most people were likely to live their entire lives in the vicinity of their birthplaces. One's parents and siblings and cousins could think of home as a single place. My father thought of home that way. The old, worn-out family farm in northern Georgia was his home. It was where his parents lived until they died and where several of his older brothers eked out a living until they, in turn, died and sons took over the barren land which they called home. For ninety-five years, nearly half the life of the United States, home to my father was one place, acting like a magnetic pole. Now the property is in strange hands, the old farmhouse abandoned and decaying.

I wonder whether there are more than a few hundred thousand people alive in the entire country who, planning to spend a few days with their parents, have that certainty *that they are going home* rather than merely to a place where their parents live. Our children will never know the intensity of such feelings; I, myself, knew that certainty only briefly. When my parents moved to a place of which I had no memories, it was no longer home. And when they moved to a retirement facility, it was only a place—not even their home.

These rooms, which I've shared with Kee, will no longer be home once she is gone. And I may find it intolerable to continue to live here. Everything will still be familiar: my body will know instinctively to turn left when leaving the bathroom, to take seven steps across the dining room to find the wall switch when it's dark, to step carefully into the hallway to avoid slipping on a throw rug. But the place will be alien to me without Kee. Had our lives been reversed, with Kee the caregiver and I the AD victim, Kee's response, I'm certain, would have been identical to mine—the numbing sense of alienation from a familiar place. The concept of home has become mobile, transient, but it is still where you love and are loved.

When our children were born, love washed over us with the force of a tsunami, leaving us clinging weakly to each other for support. As the children aged, the form and expression of that love changed, but it never shrank or dissolved; it simply took on other forms, forms more difficult to express, forms sometimes tangled with anger and disapproval as well as pride but as vibrant and demanding as when our children were conceived and emerged from Kee's womb.

Love—the ultimate romantic concept. Impossible to define, describe, or measure—neither abstract nor tangible. But I began by trying to say something about "home." Perhaps home is as mysterious as love. For me, each is melded into my union with Kee. Although I can't avoid thinking of the inevitable dissolution of our union, I do not yet understand what it will mean.

For only the second time today the telephone rings. It has to be my daughter. It's too late for a sales pitch or a casual call from a friend. Settling into a comfortable spot on the love seat, I pick up the receiver.

"Hello."

"Hi, Dad."

"I thought it had to be you. I was just getting ready to call. My grandson in bed now?"

"Well, he's in bed, but not asleep. This is one of those nights."

"Enjoy."

"Easier said than done."

"Yep, I remember; but the time will come when you'll wish you could still put him to bed rather than worrying about his not getting home when you asked him to."

"We didn't stay out terribly late."

"Ah, ah, you're being defensive, but you're right. You were pretty good about coming home as you promised. And when you were small, you gave us very little trouble going to bed. The boys were a different story. When they were small and in the same room, they gave us fits after we turned the lights off. Nothing seemed to settle them down when they had each other to torment. 'Mom, Dad—he's bothering me. I can't go to sleep.' Then we'd hear snickering and maybe a muffled voice crying out, 'He threw his pillow at me.' One of us would yell back, 'Throw it back at him and *go to sleep!*' It sounds like more fun now than it did then when we were both tired. Do you remember when you were about three or four telling your mom not to let me come when you called in the middle of the night? You had awakened feeling ill about two A.M. When you called out, I came and rocked you back to sleep—I thought. When your mom asked why you didn't want me to come you said 'Because he falls asleep when he's supposed to be rocking me.'"

"Well, you did!"

"I don't doubt it for a minute. How did your day go?"

"O.K. Nothing special but no serious problems either. I hired a new shift manager who looks very good. I'm just tired and my back has been bothering me."

"Have you been doing your exercises?"

"No, I've just been too tired at night and too rushed in the morning."

"You've got to do those exercises. If you don't, you may have to go ahead with the operation before you want to."

"I know, Dad, but sometimes. . . . How was your day?"

"Quiet. Read the paper, wrote some checks, took care of your mom. Nothing special, but I'll play golf Monday unless the weather is terrible. Do I get my grandson tomorrow?"

"That's what I'm calling about. His father has tomorrow off so they'll do something together. But next Saturday I have a morning appointment. I should be free about two. Shall I try to get a sitter for the morning, or can you manage him until I get there? What would you rather do?"

"Will you be able to stay for a while when you come? If so, I can take care of him here until you come, then Cody and I will go out and do something while you stay with your mom. I'll want to get out for a while, and I can use going wherever he wants to go as a bribe to keep him behaving in the morning. We'll manage fine. I'll just need to find out whether he'd rather go to the zoo or one of the parks. There's also a new feature at the omnimax in the science museum. He might like that, and we could hang around there until he gets tired—or I get tired. Would you like to stay for dinner—an early dinner?"

"That sounds nice. I'd like that. Can you fix something easy?"

"Haven't thought about that yet, but I can do something in the Crock-Pot. I'll just have to choose something Cody will like. That O.K.?"

"I think he'll eat whatever you decide on."

"I wouldn't bet on that, but if nothing else I can give him some hot dogs or chicken nuggets. Will he eat stir-fry now?"

"Probably not, he likes his meat in one piece."

"Well, I won't worry. We'll make out. Anyway, I'm being too much the solicitous Grumps. We didn't ask you what you wanted for supper when you were small."

"Yeah, and we had to eat all of it. What else did you do today?"

"Tonight I started to watch some television but ended up looking at some of the old slides we made on our trips. (Silence) I was trying to see if I could get any hint about when your mother's Alzheimer's became noticeable. It still bothers me that I didn't recognize it for so long."

"Dad, none of us did. We couldn't tell what was wrong. No one could. Stop blaming yourself. (Silence) Even if you had recognized it sooner, there's nothing you could have done about it. There's not much one can do now even though there are new drugs which may help in the early stages."

"I know, but it still bothers me that we kept hounding her to find something to do that would give her new interests after she quit seeing clients. I should have been able to tell that she couldn't learn to do the kinds of things we kept pushing her to do."

"Dad, I know; it bothers me, too, but . . . what else could we have done?"

"I don't know. I guess I'm just trying to unravel a ball of yarn to see what's at the center. It's silly, I guess, but still. . . . Anyway, you need to get to bed yourself. Get some sound sleep and get up in the morning early enough to do your exercises! Will we see you before next Saturday?"

"I'll come over late one afternoon, but I'm not yet sure which one."

"Wanna do lunch week after next?"

"Great. We can have a couple of hours just to talk. I'll let you know as soon as I have my schedule set."

"I'd like that."

"Dad, take care of yourself. How's your leg? I'm afraid you're trying to do too much."

"As our British friends used to say, 'Not to worry.' I'm doing O.K. Oh, by the way, I talked with your brothers t'other day and they said to give you their love."

"I really need to call them, but our schedules just don't seem to fit."

"You need to use e-mail."

"I suppose so, but I haven't gotten used to it. I'd rather talk to them. For business it's great, but I don't like to use it with people I care about—it's so—so cold, so *electronic*. Anyway, they'll be home for Christmas in a couple of months."

"Yes, and I want us to sit down together then and go over some things. I want you to begin thinking about what things here in the apartment you want, and I need to go over some financial matters all three of you need to know about, and I want to talk with all of you seriously about plans for our ashes. O.K.?"

"Yes, Dad. I know you want to do that and we will, but aren't you rushing things a bit? Just take it easy."

"To quote my loving daughter: 'Easier said than done.' But I'm quite serious about discussing our personal holdings and finances. Ashes, too! Look, you need to get to bed. I'll see you Saturday, O.K.? Love you."

"I love you, Dad. Good night."

I return the receiver to its cradle, remembering when I used to place her in her cradle—so small, so lovely, so adorable. And she still is lovely and adorable. All three of the children—so different from one another, and such a joy—well, most of the time.

Although I had planned to talk again with our children about wills, finances, and cremation at Christmas when all three will be home, I had not meant to bring it up tonight. I hadn't thought about it all day, yet there it was, popping out of my mouth. Bringing it up now, just at bedtime, was dumb, even if it did come up spontaneously.

When Kee's mother died, we followed her request to be cremated. We were afraid her sisters would disapprove, but we thought it appropriate, and the sisters at least accepted the decision. After the cremation we arranged a memorial service in her home church, then buried her ashes next to Kee's father, who had been dead for nearly thirty years. The cemetery was in the foothills of the Blue Ridge Mountains, which had been her home. Picturesque, sentimental, and right.

At the time, we agreed that we, too, would be cremated. We decided we wanted our ashes mixed and scattered to the winds from our land in Colorado. Also picturesque and sentimental, but we didn't consult the children. Funerals and bodies are for the living.

I remember all too well the first dead body I saw. I was eleven. A slightly older boy from my fifth grade class had been playing on the banks of a nearby river, fallen in, and been swept away by the current. His body was found the next day. At the funeral the family followed an old and terrible custom—an open casket in the church. I followed others in the procession past the casket. Whatever agony the drowning child felt had been erased by the mortician. The eyes were puffy and closed, his features bloated. His face was white as fresh plaster, not a hint of the lively boy I knew. Nevertheless, the swollen features conveyed the truth the mortician tried to plaster over. Silently, I swore never to look at another dead body.

Circumstances didn't allow me to keep that oath. I was present when a friend died suddenly of a heart attack. Another time I was called to the hospital to identify a colleague who, while running laps, collapsed and died of strangulation. He hadn't been carrying any identification; his glasses had been removed; and in death, his contorted face yielded no clue to his identity. I also heard my mother-in-law's body slump to the floor when her stroke came. As I struggled to move her to a bed while waiting for the ambulance, I could tell she was inert but alive, seeming only to have fainted. Before we reached the hospital, she was dead. At least I have been spared the horror of grieving over the loss of one of my children.

When Kee and I chose cremation, we did so primarily out of opposition to what has become the American ritual of death, replete with morticians' prettification, interment in waterproof, satin-lined, polished bronze caskets sealed in concrete vaults, the funeral processions, blankets of flowers, and the hushed whispers at the graveyard burial. We wanted no part of such procedures. Admittedly, I enjoy walking though old graveyards, reading into the markers narratives of grief and joy, but I now feel that money spent on funerals should be put to better use—and almost any other use is a better one.

My own mother and father lived in a community which expected funerals to be somber and monumental. Although they lived to be eighty-six and ninety-five, respectively, and were almost eager to die, I reluctantly agreed to the full treatment. What still irritates me fifteen years later is that I allowed myself to be conned by an undertaker/hustler into buying my father a new suit for burial. The body had been transported 150 miles from the retirement home to the mortuary clad only in a nightshirt. All of his clothes remained at the home. Even though the casket was to remain closed, the mortician insisted on a cheap suit, and I collapsed before the force of tradition. Disgusting. The dignity of simplicity strangled by intertwined cords of tradition and false religious sentiment. Assuming Peter and the Golden Gate, the first conversation would be about cheap fabric.

In spite of my objections to common burial rites, I recognize the importance of ceremony to the grief process. Kee wrote on grief and trained counselors to deal specifically with those who, having lost infants, were encouraged by hospitals, churches, and communities to deny their grief. She told of one mother who, having experienced neonatal death, was approached by a nurse who assured her that her baby was in heaven. She blurted out, "I don't want my baby in heaven. I want her in my arms." Some of Kee's understanding may have rubbed off on me.

Neither of us wants to be memorialized in concrete or marble. Yet I don't want our passing to go by like a blip disappearing from a radar screen. I want our children to have ample opportunity to develop those ceremonies of loss which most serve their needs. But what? They would have to mingle the ashes; they would have to make the journey to Colorado. What do they want? I must talk that through with them—and soon.

Customs for the disposal of the human body have always fascinated me: the funeral pyres of the Indian subcontinent, a genuine ritual of grief, but absurd in the context of American life; the custom of some American Indian tribes long ago of placing bodies on platforms exposed to the elements, a custom fitting to their understanding of life, but inconceivable now even in Colorado or Montana; the simplicity and affirmation of grief expressed in Orthodox Judaism with its quick disposition of the body in a simple wooden coffin. Or Swift's description of burial customs in Lilliput, where bodies were buried vertically, head down so that in the next world they would land on their feet. That probably catches the uniqueness of such practices best of all. To one not a part of the culture, burial procedures are alien and humorous. To one immersed in the culture, no other option seems sensible. Kee and I find ancient mummification and modern cryogenics equally appalling. Dust to dust, ashes to ashes is our choice, but will that choice serve the children? I want them to know our preference, but they should make the decision.

One thing that my daughter said amuses me. She prefers the telephone to e-mail. She is her mother's daughter. Kee, too, liked the telephone, preferring to hear the inflections, tones, even pauses occurring in conversation—matters concealed by the flatness of letters or e-mail. And it's certainly true that something charged with meaning in speech can seem quite innocuous and trite on paper or screen. The dismissal of e-mail as being "so electronic" doesn't dismiss its usefulness, however. As for the telephone, when we were talking, we expressed so little of what we felt. I didn't pour out the depth of my affection for her or my dependence on Cody for a sense of vitality and enthusiasm, and, yes, commitment to the future. I didn't even tell Kristin how grateful I was that she called me, nor did I say that each call from our sons is worth a thousand times its cost. How could I?

My next thought is "How could I not?" Thinking of our children sustains me through Kee's illness. When they visit, they are my comforters. Yet what do I say to them? "Thank you for coming. It's meant a great deal to me." Yecch! It distresses me that the deeper the feeling, the harder it is to give voice to it.

Years ago I was asked to give the eulogy at the funeral of a dear friend, a woman who was Kee's best friend. I began the eulogy with a colloquial phrase: "What's to say? It's not that words are inadequate. Anne loved language. It does not behoove us to spurn anything she loved. The problem is that I can't find the right words." I still feel that way. Sometime, somehow I must find the words that will begin to express to our children some portion of what they meant and mean to us. But words are so entangled in the guts of feeling that they can't be dragged out without sounding maudlin. Or is that it? What's wrong with allowing sentiment to gain full expression? Maybe what I fear is that dragging the words out of my guts will make me feel naked, exposed, defenseless.

Sophistication and love, I think, are mortal enemies. The more clinically aware one is of human relations and the more one knows about biological needs and social dependencies, the harder it is to believe in love. Once, talking with some students informally, I said that love cannot be analyzed or submitted to tests. Any effort to place it on an examining table changes and violates it. What is being examined becomes only the residue of what it once was. At the time I rather liked the metaphor, and still think it conveys something of the mystery of love, but it doesn't go far enough, and maybe it even goes in the wrong direction by making love an object.

I know I never adequately conveyed to my parents my love for them or convinced them that I admired them in spite of our differences. Oh, I used the right words—sometimes—but that intense, deep-seated feeling for them called love I could never adequately convey. With Kee I think I succeeded better, verbally and physically. Even where our interests diverged, as with golf, we came to respect the other's preferences. More important, we came to love being with the other, and touch was central to our sharing.

With her illness, intercourse became less frequent and then stopped altogether. Perhaps Kee might have enjoyed the intimacy, but as her physical response decreased, I felt that penetrating her was a violation of our relationship, something closer to masturbation. After her falls, intercourse would only have caused her pain. This is difficult to talk about. It involves the greatest intimacy we can know, and intimacy, too, escapes language, degenerating into discussion of erotic stimulation and alternative positions. I don't think that's equivalent to love, although ignorance of both may generate hatred.

Intercourse and love sometimes have little in common. We know that violence can be a part of the act, and if it predominates there is no love, only the satisfaction of physical release or dominance. Nor can love making be an act of sympathy. Sharing love through intercourse, through becoming one for a brief time, rhythmically united and seeking each other's pleasure, is only one form of love, but ecstatic beyond all other experience. One doesn't "make love." One discovers and shares it. I hope that our children have a partial sense of the intensity of our physical feeling for one another. I'm afraid I have never been able to imagine my parents taking any pleasure in intercourse. Over the last few years of Kee's illness what has meant most to both of us is the simple pat or nudge, the taking hold of hands and squeezing, the kiss on the forehead or nape of the neck. Even my indifferent success in brushing her hair duplicates the strokes of a lover. The physical is never unimportant. That is most evident if, in lifting Kee from the wheelchair to place her in bed, I slip and half drop her on the bed. She looks up in alarm, not from pain, I think, but from fear that I am angry. Once the rug slipped beneath me as I put her down, and I fell on top of her. A quick "Wups, I slipped—but since I'm here I think I'll stay" brought a smile, almost a laugh.

Kee also responds warmly to terms of endearment. Calling her by name means less than "love" or "sweetie." The important thing is her association with the words. One word in particular gives her pleasure—"snuggery." We called our land in Colorado "The Aerie"—a high nesting place. When we moved to this condo on the tenth floor, one of us used the word *snug* and from it came "Snuggery" as the name for our new home. I looked the word up in a dictionary and found it to be synonymous with "aerie"—a lucky hit. From the beginning she liked the word and its connotations. Any use of "Snuggery" gives her reassurance. My one slip in mentioning a nursing home when I was most depressed has not been repeated. To lose her "Snuggery" while I am alive would wound her deeply.

I still have things to do before going to bed. To do or not to do my exercises is no longer at issue. The need to maintain some degree of strength and agility so that I can care for Kee is essential. My back injury and the devastation of my left leg force me to work hard to maintain the little strength I have. Get off the treadmill and the generator stops.

Like so much else in my life, exercises are done because they must be done. I find no pleasure in them. The exercises aren't demanding, but finding the will to do them at any time is difficult. My innate tendency to postpone, hoping that whatever problem I'm facing will simply disappear, is always present. "Oh, I'll wait and do them tomorrow when I'm feeling stronger" is the self-deceit I have to fight against every night.

The exercises are designed to strengthen back, abdomen, leg, and neck muscles. It's too late to worry about biceps. When I had the shingles and was deeply depressed, a physical therapist asked me how I could drive. I was dumbfounded. She pointed out that I could turn my head only a few degrees. How, she asked, did I look over my left shoulder when entering intersections? My response, "Very carefully," did not amuse her. So she had me begin a series of exercises to strengthen and loosen the neck muscles constricted by arthritis and to improve my increasingly turtlelike posture. Do you remember Walt Kelly? A genius! I don't want to look like Pogo's friend, Turtle. Well . . . retaining a shell for emergency use may have its advantages.

The neck exercise involves sitting up straight against a wall, pressing the skull and neck as far back as I can and gradually turning my head left, then right, each time striving to turn my chin farther and farther toward the shoulder. It can be painful. The other exercises involve lying on the floor, lifting and stretching legs while scrunching my abdomen, and raising my knees to my chest. I can do them all in about twenty minutes. The deterrent is inertia. Why bother? Do I really want to get down on the floor when I get so dizzy trying to get back up? Who needs it? I do.

While I do my exercises, I usually listen to CNN, but tonight I choose a local station's late news. I can't watch the screen steadily, but that's rarely necessary. Tonight the top story is a fire that swept through a two-story house in the early evening. An anchorman summarizes the tragedy; footage of the fire gutting the house plays, then there is a shot of smoldering ruins. An on-site reporter gives the location and, with a grim expression, states that a mother and her three children have died of smoke inhalation. The camera switches to firemen bringing the bodies out of the rubble.

I know what's coming next, having seen such coverage all too often. The camera zooms in on a soot-smeared fireman. An unseen reporter thrusts a microphone in the fireman's face and makes a statement posed as a question: "You were one of those who brought the bodies out."

"Yes."

"Were the bodies badly burned?"

"No."

The reporter pauses, seeking a more profitable line of questioning.

"Can you tell us where the bodies were found?"

"They were near the stairwell on the second floor."

"Huddled together or separately?"

"Together."

"What position were they in?"

"The mother was holding the baby. The older children were next to her."

"Is this one of the worst fires you've seen?"

And so it continues, the reporter milking the scene for pathos, the fireman, to his credit, answering tersely with increasing irritation. I want the fireman to knock the microphone away or, better yet, knock the reporter down. There is another close-up of the mother's sister, who is hysterical and cannot answer questions.

The program cuts back to the anchorman who says, "And now to our sports reporter. Harry, what do you have for us tonight?"

There was a time when I would have been sufficiently outraged to call the station then follow up with a letter. How anyone can intrude on victims or heroes with such obscene questions surpasses my understanding. The station would claim it was just trying to provide the "inside" story to its viewers. But no inside story is presented, and the reporters are capitalizing on the sensational with no concern for the privacy of victims or their families. Now I'm tired, weary of the insensitivity, weary of false justifications, weary of my frustrations.

Before long, reporters and their intrusive cameras will be camping on a neighbor's lawn grilling a teenager. "We understand that your mother has uterine cancer. Is that true?"

"Yes."

"Would you tell us how you feel about that?"

I turn off the television and finish my exercises in silence, grumbling to myself not only about insensitivity, but also about what passes for news—beautiful people with immaculate coiffures and cosmetic teeth shifting on cue from tragic masks to comic masks. Six minutes for sponsors, four for the weather, five for sports, six for local stories, three to four minutes pretending to be intimate friends, perhaps four minutes for national or world events—if time permits. Am I the only crank out here in TV Land?

Sitting on the floor until some brief dizziness passes, I hug my knees. I've already dismissed my disgust with the "news" and still feel warm from the chat with Kristin. I give my knees an extra squeeze. It's not the embrace I prefer. Getting up is slow and painful. "Dem bones, dem bones gonna walk around." The old spiritual is a kind of resurrection theme. Usually I substitute "gotta" for "gonna."

Now to confront the momentous decision as to whether apple or grapefruit juice will be my nightcap. Why take either? Habit, I guess. Opening the refrigerator door I find the apple juice blocking my path to the grapefruit juice. Has fate's unseen hand edged the apple juice in front of the grapefruit? Of course not. I remember now holding the apple juice bottle just a while ago. Obstinately, I declare for the grapefruit juice. I am as much the master of my fate as William Ernest Henley, poor soul.

On the shelf below, there are two packages of cookies—pecan shortbreads and chocolate wafers—more choices. The shortbread is already open. Perhaps an aching, insatiable desire for chocolate could tempt me to struggle with more plastic, but I pick up two shortbread cookies and head for my study where I sip the juice and nibble at the cookies while thinking that tomorrow will bring more of the same. Then I remember the day's three washes and spend twenty minutes smoothing and sorting sheets, clothes, and towels.

Time for yet another ritual. Brushing my teeth is as essential as doing the exercises. Gingivitis led to surgical procedures on my gums and ultimately to titanium implants. I have lost more teeth than I can remember, but the marvels of modern dentistry have produced bridges and implants which have staved off the necessity of turning to dental plates, which were the fate of both my mother and father. Where was fluoride when we needed it?

For a number of years I've used an electric toothbrush, so delightful a toy that my grandson enjoys using it when he sleeps over. The whirring of the motor and the vibration of the bristles make him laugh. A good combination—pleasure in the pursuit of insidious bacteria. Few of the boy's struggles against destructive forces will give him such pleasure. Let him enjoy while he can. I don't get the same pleasure but settle for a necessary job carefully done.

Cleaning the brush and returning it to its base, I glance once more into the old mirror. The mirror caught me off balance this morning. Now it reflects a familiar face unperturbed at the moment by questions of identity. Unfortunately—or perhaps fortunately—I look as old as I did this morning, maybe a wee bit older. The preacher in Ecclesiastes is right. Aging is a steady, inexorable process. When we are young, we cannot imagine being old. We watch our parents and their friends. In aunts and uncles whom we see infrequently we can better mark the deepening wrinkles and halting movements, even the occasional vacancy of the eyes. But observing the aging of others is of a different dimension than coming to terms with our own aging. We admit that we can no longer run as fast as we once did but feed our self-image by noting those few things we can do better than when we were swift youths. We know that aging is occurring moment by moment, and we call it maturing. We avert our face from awareness that ripening is a process that ends in rotting. Even now, I have difficulty accepting that simple greengrocer's fact. Awareness of the inexorable passage of the human form from birth to dissolution lies buried deeply in human consciousness. We sense the tremors which weaken the foundation of our lives but wilfully ignore the rumblings, the certainty of what is to come.

You find that observation too negative? Why? It has its own beauty. We are part of the natural order. In aging and decaying we're true to nature's fixed pattern. Would you want it any other way? I wouldn't . . . yet diseases and dementia seem to me to violate the process of aging. What I fear is not death, but the loss of awareness.

A poem of Yeats delights me:

> An aged man is but a paltry thing,
> A tattered coat upon a stick, unless
> Soul clap its hands and sing, and louder sing
> For every tatter in its mortal dress.

I want to celebrate rather than lament blemishes and imperfections. To celebrate being human may be the noblest act any of us can perform.

Even the imperfections of our society and the human sadness we find around us are, I believe, counterpointed by beauty and goodness. When the bumper sticker "Shit Happens" was popular, I thought about producing one that read "So Does Beauty!"

Most of my life I've tried to sing, even to let my soul clap hands joyfully. But now that's hard—with Kee as she is. God, I miss her.

On my way to the bedroom, I pause before the living room window. Beyond the sparse light from the park is the glow of the city. Hospitals, court buildings, skyscrapers which house banks and insurance companies, all are illuminated against the night sky. The lights of a plane in its landing pattern arc across the sky, the plane's passengers intent on their destination. Beneath them their fellow men pursue individual courses in apartment buildings, houses, and the few businesses or factories still open. I stand apart but as one of them. Out there are other victims of disease and with them, if they are fortunate, their own caregivers. We form a too silent community. The poor among us have virtually no voice at all.

Particularly do I sympathize with caregivers who, late in life and perhaps in ill health, must assist a spouse with Alzheimer's. Lacking the resources, the health, the strength essential to the caregiver, how can they possibly cope? If there is no money to hire aides, if family members can give little help, if they depend on what little they get from Medicare or Medicaid, they live out a tragedy beyond my comprehension. I find it odd to think so, but I am one of the more fortunate.

For a long time I have wondered how to raise public consciousness about the plight of those with low incomes who are stricken with dementia. As yet, I have done nothing about it except sympathize, and that is not enough. We need to develop more concerted action groups to raise public consciousness of the need to provide public funds to assist needy families suffering through dementia. Without public pressure, there will be insufficient help forthcoming from government or health agencies.

Some of our friends thought Kee's activity on behalf of the Committee for a SANE Nuclear Policy in the 1950s was hopeless, but who knows the consequences of what she and others like her did? The bombs were not dropped! She would want me to try to effect change. Maybe people will awaken to the need as the number who suffer grows. I have to get myself together. I have to try, and the place to begin is the local Alzheimer's Association.

In the bedroom, in faint light, I slip into pajamas. The sheet is wrapped around Kee. As gently as I can, I pull it out from under her and stretch it over to my side of the bed, fluff the pillow slightly, and prepare to climb in. When Kee began to go to bed early, I gave up reading in bed and even moved the small compact television out of the bedroom.

Tonight I sense that I am leaving something undone. Some sense of omission bothers me. There is no dog or cat to put out or take in. Our last dog died twelve years ago, and the last cat soon thereafter. I know that on my way from the bathroom to the bedroom, I checked the lights. All were off except the one on a timer. No unwanted utilities are on. There is something else.

Briefly I review my day. My brain buzzed constantly, bouncing about, nosing into closets, poking holes in fabrics, keeping me distraught and uneasy. I know my irritability and my silly soliloquies are merely attempts to come to terms with the continuing stress and my many failures during this ordeal.

It's a useless review. I try to frame the overarching question. Something is wrong with the way I'm attempting to understand our plight. I'm trying to impose a design on life, and I can't complete the pattern. As in a crossword puzzle, I am trying to fill in spaces where I can't find a word or phrase synonymous with the clue, or I've made guesses that are simply wrong. Letting go of the urgent need to understand may be the hardest thing I ever do, yet I think I have to let go. If there is a pattern, it's beyond my understanding. I can neither determine what it is nor unravel it. It's simply there.

When I was a small boy, one of my parents, usually my mother, said prayers with me every night. I didn't kneel by the side of the bed as shown in children's books of the time. Rather, lying snugly in bed with a comforting hand holding mine, I prayed, "God, bless Momma, God bless Daddy, bless my brother, and bless me and help me to do Thy Will." It was a simple prayer and probably more mechanical repetition than prayer. But seventy years later, I can't improve on it even if I disbelieve that anyone knows precisely what the will of God is. Three of those upon whom I then sought blessings have been dead for years. I alone remain in the flesh, susceptible to the temptations of the flesh, but particularly susceptible to anger, sometimes greed, and above all arrogance.

Arrogance has driven me all day. I want to know precisely when signs of Kee's affliction began, to know why I did not detect what signs there were. Even the question whether I've done my very best to care for her and to express my love for her is unanswerable. When I try to peer into mind and soul to know whether I am truly grateful that I am able, physically and financially, to care for her, I find half-truths everywhere; versions of yes and no plague every question.

Like Job I scream for understanding. "Why was my wife afflicted with Alzheimer's disease?" The answers of the "comforters" haven't improved appreciably over the millennia. Job's demands and lamentations are not answered; they are silenced by the vision of the mysterious, creative power of ISNESS. "I AM WHAT I AM"; "I WILL BE WHAT I WILL BE." The ultimate enigma. The unsolvable puzzle. Maybe like Job I've been plodding toward that recognition, toward the reality that there is no explanation.

When as a child I said my prayers, I suppose I thought of God as a powerful, kindly, and generous old grandfather. Since my own grandfathers died before I was born, they couldn't threaten that image. If I visualized what God looked like, I must have seen him as a less portly Santa Claus with a little less twinkle in his eye.

Now I am drawn to the Jewish conviction that the name of divinity is too sacred to be pronounced. The Tetragrammaton represents a mystery beyond human ken. The icons we make are a substitute for the speechless awe that the sacred demands. I was taught that taking the name of God in vain is blasphemous. Now I look on those who profess to have an intimate knowledge of divinity and who claim to speak on behalf of divinity as the ones who are truly blasphemous.

I cannot put into words what I believe. Words, too, are part of a man-made design to understand and to control. When I worship, expressing adoration and praise, when, with varying degrees of success, I try to be receptive to what I think is best in life, I do so in a vortex which sucks up all the creeds which make God in man's image. The human need to make *MYSTERY* familiar and comfortable speaks poignantly to human limitations.

In my late teens, I believed I had a mission to perform, a vocation, but didn't know what it was. It was a long time before I decided to become a teacher. After I did, most of my waking hours were devoted to preparing for and performing what I think to be the mission of any good teacher: to know those facts and procedures that are knowable and to teach them urgently; to open minds to possibilities; to encourage thoughtfulness, thoroughness, and honesty, above all with oneself; to learn to synthesize experience and incorporate it into a personal, integral, ethical design; to develop the intellectual and emotional balance that enables one to confront creatively the turbulence and change inevitable in life; to view life with awe and joy; to pursue any course generously and compassionately.

That I chose to teach literature was almost accidental. I could have pursued the same sense of mission by teaching history, biology, political science, or any discipline. It wasn't even necessary to become a teacher. I could have pursued the same mission in sales or plumbing, in law, medicine, or the arts. I now believe that what I considered to be my mission is not at all distinctive. It's the mission of mankind. In absolute terms, we are all doomed to failure, but each partial accomplishment is in itself a triumph.

Maybe my vocation as teacher prepared me inadequately for my new vocation. By nature and training, I fear, I am unsuited to the often praised tranquil acceptance of the caregiver. I want explanations, and there are none. When I try to be a model of patience, I can't be. When I try to be "positive" about Kee's condition, I find it impossible. Never have I engaged in any other struggle which I knew to be utterly lost from the beginning.

Even if I were "perfect," the ideal giver of care, I would fail. There is no way known to science or magic to overcome Kee's affliction. That her dementia will end in death does not distress me. To be born is to die. Death in an accident or from cancer or pneumonia would have left me grief stricken but, I think, not so weary and confused. Friends who were dying in agony from cancer or ALS retained consciousness and intelligence. As far as I can tell, my wife long ago surrendered the important human faculties, except, I hope, the supreme capacity, the capacity to love.

Standing by the bed my wife has honored, I pray, not as a child, but as an aging, tired, confused old man. The words aren't voiced and are only partially formed in my mind, but I pray that I can relinquish my desperate need to know and understand, accepting what was and is with courage and grace. I pray that I might live to serve my children and grandchild and as many others as I can who live under the canopy of darkness. I pray that I might counter Santayana's half-truthful observation that life is a predicament by insisting that there is also joy in life, a joy I have known with my wife and through my wife. Finally, I pray for all those attempting to combat Alzheimer's and the other diseases consuming mankind, for those striving to assist and comfort primary caregivers, for those who are and will become primary caregivers. May they survive their suffering creatively.

Kee is snoring—short, hiccupy snorts. I climb into bed beside her and reach over and touch her. I lie here thinking that tomorrow will be like today, combining the same duties, the same opportunities, the same irritations, the same gentle woman whom I love, the same irascible, confused, self-doubting me. I don't really want it any other way.

I didn't draw the blinds before lying down. The lights of the city are diffuse but strong enough to cast a slight shadow on the ceiling. In the semidarkness, I see the shadow of our canopy and know that it is still imperfect. Somehow, to sleep below it is comforting.

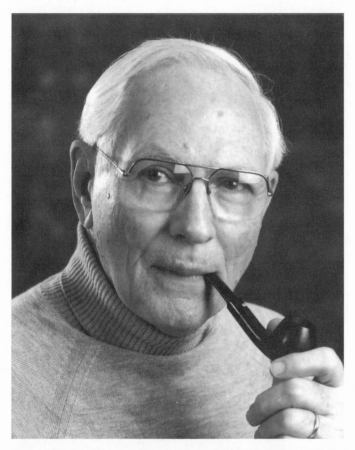

Burton M. Wheeler is Professor Emeritus of English and Religious Studies at Washington University in St. Louis, Missouri. He served as Dean of the College of Arts and Science from 1966 to 1978 and Interim Dean of Libraries from 1988 to 1989.